MUSCLE MIND

MUSCLE MIND

—

CHANGE YOUR MIND
CHANGE YOUR BODY
CHANGE YOUR LIFE

Robert Grant

How Developing a Method of Thinking Can Offer
Success in Any Goal in Life

ISBN: 197381126X
ISBN 13: 9781973811268
Library of Congress Control Number: 2017911544
CreateSpace Independent Publishing Platform
North Charleston, South Carolina

INTRODUCTION

This book is dedicated to you. Yes, you. Because I was once you. Looking for help. Help in navigating myself and my life. By choosing to read this book, you are proving you have already started the process of realizing your full potential. This book is my way of giving my little bit back to the world. I want to share my experience and struggles with as many people as possible, in hopes that it may help others realize that it is within them, within everyone, to reach their definition of success in life. I was able to teach myself a method of thinking that I developed through weight training and have applied to my entire life. This way of thinking allows me to reach the goals I set in front of myself. I want to share this with others, to help them do the same. Determine what you want, write it down, and look at it every day. This thinking method is not just for the gym; it can be applied to all aspects of life and utilized to acquire your greatest desire and to conquer each of your goals along the way to your greatest success.

Greatness exists within you. It is there. Deep down inside of you, somewhere, someone other than who you are right now exists. You must only find the purpose in your life that is worth changing for. You must focus on your thought process that has been programmed for you by your environment up until now. Have the courage to show that other person. Show the person you know you really are to the world. Don't let anyone stop you. Keep your mind focused on your vision of what happiness is for you. You only have one life. Let's get started. You're already behind schedule.

HAVE YOU HIT ROCK BOTTOM?

I MADE THE mistake early in life of doing what I thought others approved of me doing, instead of doing what I desired for myself. I picked a path that I believed would earn the respect of my family and of my spouse, while providing a modest wage, instead of creating the lifestyle I truly wanted. I once believed in my youth that asserting yourself with boisterous anger and aggressiveness was a sign of power. However, naturally I was a calm and reserved individual, so I believed I was somehow inferior, since it was not in my nature to intimidate or show anger or hostility.

Later in life, I would realize that my natural poise and self-control would constitute much more power and dominance than any fit of rage or show of aggression. This comes from our society showing a steady stream of aggression and violence through media and entertainment sources like news, TV shows, movies, and music. The aggressive, dominant male is always shown as the hero and the example of the paramount male aim.

Studying the influences that are viewed by young males in their upbringing would show why such assumptions where made in my case and ultimately shaped my decision making. The male roles are often aggressive, alpha-male individuals who earned respect by taking it either through intimidation or violence. The belief that in order to be a man of a certain caliber I needed to attain a certain level of aggressiveness led me into a job field that would surely develop those attitudes I held in high regard and thought that others held in just as high a regard.

This was not who I was. I was trying to be someone I thought society held in high regard. I thought that in order to be a man of a certain stature, like the ones I saw depicted in film and listened to in music, I would have to develop a hard-nosed, mean, and cold personality. This went against everything I was naturally. Two of my major employers were the Canadian military and the Ministry of Corrections. So, needless to say, putting myself in a law-enforcement environment for years of my life eventually saddened me to the point where I was forced by health complications to take time to reflect on who I was, what I was doing, the people I was around every day, how it was influencing me, how it was affecting my health and the health of my relationships, and how I was going to change it. I had to change it if I were to have a hope of living in true happiness.

This decision came to pass one night, having just lain down to sleep. My two dogs, my spouse, and I lay there half awake. I remember my thoughts being very intense and rushing through my mind faster than I had ever experienced. Two days before this, at work, I had witnessed a man die of a drug overdose; the same day as I lay there in my bed, I witnessed a man grab another by the back of the head and proceed to smash it repeatedly off a metal windowsill until the victim was lifeless. Such sadness I felt for the lives that were being wasted in that place. Ultimately, it wasn't the violence I had witnessed or the threat of violence toward me that was disturbing me so greatly. It was the thought of being trapped working in that negative, dark, and dysfunctional environment for the rest of my working days. This thinking brought on a wave of panic and sparked the first anxiety attack I had ever experienced.

I felt like I could no longer control my thoughts; they were out of control. I felt as if someone were squeezing the air out of my lungs, and I was almost certain I was going to die. I felt like at any moment, I was going to scream for help uncontrollably. I rolled to my side on one elbow to try to catch my breath, and my movement stirred my spouse. She asked me what I was doing. It was all I could muster with all my mind and body to whisper, "I am all right; I'm OK," so as not to scare her into a panic. I eventually stood myself up and managed to walk to the front door of my house. I went outside and sat down on the front steps in my underwear, trying to control my thoughts and my breathing.

I remember clutching my cell phone and trying to bring up the dial pad, since I was sure I was going to have to call 911. It was November, definitely below zero degrees Celsius, and here I was, thinking, *I'm going to die in my underwear on my front steps*, from something I didn't even understand at the time. Eventually, though, the cold air cooled me down; I was able to regain my breath and began to try to decipher what had just happened to me. This was when I knew change was inevitable. It wasn't until six months after that experience that loss of consciousness due to high blood pressure pointed out to me that I had no choice. It was time to change. I decided I needed to get back to who I knew I really was. I was not cold; I was not hard or aggressive; I did not want to be involved in conflict and violence on a daily basis. These were not who I was inside, though I did learn I *can* be those things if I need to be, but they are not fundamentally how I wanted to go through life. I looked back on my life and realized I had the ability to imagine anything in the world I wanted to become and the character to make it happen. Instead, I allowed the suggestions of others and the influence of society in general to shape my thoughts, rather than following what I knew to be true of myself. No one is going to dream a dream for you.

Only you know what you want to become. It takes thought. Think hard about what makes you feel happy. What gives you purpose and makes you feel fulfilled? What would you want your life to look like if you could have it any way you wanted? What are your *musts*? When I was in school, everyone would always ask, "What do you want to be?" and well, I wish someone would have asked, "Who are you already?" The trick is you need to know yourself incredibly well. Dream what you desire, and take action moving toward that every day. Do not take a job just for the money. Do not work a job that gives you no fulfillment. If you are just getting through your day on a daily basis, you are just getting through your life. What kind of life is that? That is no life I want any part of. But the line of work I chose because I desired to be in it. My desires, however, were not formed properly. I desired it for the wrong reasons. I could have desired anything and brought that desire into existence, but instead I chose based on the opinions of others. So set your goals and desires high. Stay away from influences that distract you from your dreams, and stay focused on what you truly want. Strive for it like your life depends on it, because *it does*!

———

TAKE CONTROL

YOUR LIFE IS all your own. It is completely within your control. The world paints an illusion that this is not true. The sooner you realize this fact, the sooner you can start to achieve your dreams; the sooner you can realize your potential. Everyone is a marvelous creation of energy from the same source. We are all connected in space and time by the same universal substance. Science is proving this true. If you want proof, research string theory and quantum entanglement. Somewhere inside your mind, you know who you were really meant to be. You may not think so right now, but that person is there, waiting for you to discover him or her. There is a saying that "The mighty oak must first live within the acorn." This is the belief and acknowledgment that we are all like the acorn. The acorn is birthed from the mighty oak tree, dropped into an environment, the soil, and to what height and health it grows is based on what the acorn absorbs from its environment.

You have to get to a point where you are able to think as the person you wish to become would think. Act the way that person would act. That vision of who you want to be in your mind—think how that person would act in the situation you are currently stuck in. You can't expect to get to be that person, going out for dinner four times a week and ordering whatever he or she wants on the menu and expect to have your dream physique. The same way you can't spend eight hours of your day playing video games and watching nonsense on the TV and then expect to be a CEO. You have to be willing to sacrifice the person you are for the person you want to become. If you are OK with the life you have, eating whatever you want and wasting time on TV and video games, that's fine. Just don't expect to have the life that comes from not wasting time and having discipline, and don't complain about other people not choosing what you have chosen. You lie in the bed you make for yourself. You can't complain that yours is messy if you don't take the time to make it.

Part of becoming successful is discovering the person you were truly meant to be, free from the paradigm that has been pushed upon you by your environment up until now. Aristotle said, "Know thyself." You need to think of how you are smart—not how much smarter you are than anyone else. Forget competition. Competition is an affirmation of scarcity and fear. You need to find how you are smart, what you are good at, and what excites you. What is important to you. This is the only way to know how you truly want to live your life. Health and fitness are only one small aspect of a life that is full of bliss and joy. There are many other aspects that make up a happy and fulfilling life. To be fully fulfilled in life, you must reach your full potential in all areas. Figure out your strengths. Ask yourself how your strengths are valuable. Think every day about being successful using what you are good at or what you have a genuine interest in. What sparks your curiosity? How can you use that to better the lives of the people around you? Through knowing that, you will start your path to finding wealth and happiness.

Life is full of many ups and downs, and everyone goes through immense turmoil. There are endless distractions and negative events that take place in every life. The difference in achieving steps toward your success or reverting back down the stairs you have already climbed is your ability to react in a way that favors your goals. You must look at what is happening in your life and be able to see those situations as an outside observer. Acknowledge that this negative instance is happening, be it a negative person, the loss of a job or lack thereof, emotional strain from a romantic relationship, or a death in the family. The circumstance may not be in your control, *but* your reaction to the situation most definitely is. If you can train your mind to react in your favor, instead of allowing your thoughts to spiral out of control, you will succeed in anything you set out to do. You have to force yourself to be a master of your own emotions. This is one of the most powerful skills to develop in the human mind.

> The people will not revolt. They will not look up from their screens long enough to notice what's happening.
> —George Orwell, 1949

There are many distractions in this world, some of which are there purposely. Television, Facebook, advertising, cellphones, email, car radio—all of these provide noise in your daily environment. Some are there as a part of your home environment: pets, laundry, dishes, kids, and yardwork are all distractions. Weather, other drivers, and the general public are all forms of distraction. The better you are at selecting what information enters your mind, the more control you have over it. In order to get more in tune with your mind and your body, you need to silence all of this outside noise. You need to control what you think and how you feel on a daily basis. This means getting rid of all the negative information you are allowing your mind to absorb. Turn off the TV, or at least watch something that is supportive of your goals. Do not pay attention to the news; it has zero benefit to you. Think, if you did not watch the news for the last ten years of your life, would you have lived your life any differently? Not likely, though you definitely would have had a more peaceful, serene state of mind. I could never, for the life of me, understand why anyone would watch the news first thing in the morning. The news is simply informing you of all the negative things that have happened in the world in the last twenty-four hours. Instead of the news, turn on a motivational speech, turn on some uplifting positive music, or read an uplifting book.

That information is poisonous to anyone who is trying to reach success. Flood your mind with positivity. If you live in a house where the yardwork takes up five hours of your day three times a week and it's stopping you from having time to work on what you really want to work on, you may want to consider downsizing. You have to be aware of what it limiting your time and your mind. If you spend all your time in the car, listening to music you aren't really interested in, mixed with radio advertisements trying to control your choices, that's wasting your time and your mind. Instead, you may consider listening to audiobooks or download instructional videos or motivational speeches from your computer and listen to them instead. Control your environment. That time you spend with your mind unfocused is time you could be using more wisely.

Maintaining a positive state of mind keeps you grateful for the good in the world and vice versa. It creates a positive vibration in your soul that can be felt by everyone who comes in contact with you. If you are sour and bitter at what is happening in the world, regardless of whether it has any impact on you at all, and you go out into the general public and interact with others, I guarantee you that your interactions will be different than if you went out and felt good about who you are and the good things life has given you, and be hopeful and happy, knowing you are working on your success. That positivity can be felt, and it will be passed on to everyone you come in contact with.

If you allow people and situations to take you out of that state of mind, you are allowing those thoughts to control you. You must accept that negative things do happen. That is part of life in this world, but your reaction to it can be within your control. If you are emotionally controlled by the world, you will never get to where you need to be mentally. Think of when you were a child and you asked your parents for something like candy or a toy at the store, and they told you no. Then you cried and perhaps were disciplined. The candy is stimulating emotion within you of *wanting*, and the denial of the candy by your parents is stimulating the reaction of frustration, sadness, anger, and resentment. When you stop this reactive state of mind and learn to control your emotions, you instantly grow into a stronger person and are elevated to a higher consciousness. This is what your parents developed in you, or what you as a parent are developing in your child when you say no. This is why kids are said to be *spoiled* when parents give in to their children too often. The children never learn to develop this skill of controlling their emotions when life doesn't go their way. This can result later in life in relationship issues, poor financial-management practices, and conflict with authority. This is why the majority of children who are raised in foster care or have grown up with very little parenting often end up in the criminal-justice system. They simply failed to develop proper emotional reactions to unfavorable instances in life.

Practice catching yourself thinking negatively, and the quicker you can get yourself back to being happy and grateful for what you have, regardless of what others are thinking, saying, and doing, the more progress you will make toward your success, and the shorter your battle will be. If you can master your emotions, it will add an immense amount of personal power and confidence into your life. This is a vital aspect of achieving your goals and dreams. If you are always allowing negativity to influence your mind, you will never reach your full potential. So much of success is based on personal

mental fortitude and discipline. If you are always allowing outside influences to tell you what to think, instead
of trusting yourself and pushing toward your goals, you
will never get there.

Every day, I see people at the gym watching the news
while they are working out, or watching a TV show or
texting people. To me, this shows an incredible lack
of focus on their goals and what they wish to achieve.
Those are the same people who will come up to me and
ask me if I am on steroids, since there is obviously no
way I could be in such great shape without them. Well,
you know what? When I am on the treadmill or in the
gym, I do not watch the rubbish that is placed in front
of me on that TV screen. The first thing I do is shut it
off. I will walk at a good pace with my eyes closed for a
while and just escape into my own mind. I remind myself why I am there. I think of my goals and where I want
to be. I visualize the life I want. I visualize what this
work is doing to my body. I will turn on a motivational
speech and listen to it while I push myself way out of my
comfort zone. I force positive thoughts upon my mind
by reciting affirmations that maintain my focus on what
I want and who I want to be. My mental state is totally
elevated to be focused, grateful, and positive while I am
pushing myself to be better every day. No steroid in the
world will change your thoughts to what you need them
to be. Only you can do that. If you want something that

the majority of people don't have, you need to do what the majority of people aren't willing to do.

You need to elevate your mind above the normal plane of thinking. Stop being subject to what the world would have you believe. Stop being told what to think, and don't be afraid to think differently than everyone else. If you think the same way everyone else thinks, there is only one option: to get the results everyone else has. Look around you, and see who you surround yourself with. Which of them are influencing your thoughts? If you are around dark and negative people all day long, day in and day out, guess what? You are absorbing all of that negativity into your mind. My grandfather told me once, if you roll with the pigs, you're going to get covered in shit. It took me the majority of my adolescence to come to terms with what he meant by this. You need to find the people who are going to be an asset to your thinking. Seek out others who are on the same path, those people who have the same goals and are pushing to reach the same state of mind and body you are. If you have a goal of building a race car, why would you hang out around people who are building doghouses?

RE-PROGRAM YOUR MIND

You have been programmed by your environment since the day you were born. All you have done since birth is absorb information. Negative or positive, everything you now know, think, feel, or believe, you have absorbed from outside sources. In order to elevate your mind, you need to develop your own beliefs, thoughts, and feelings. Know where you want to go, who you want to be, what you want to look like, and how you want to live. Know it without hesitation. Visualize it every day. Know it like you know the back of your hand. Think about it every day. Shut out the outside influence, and hold these wants in your thoughts all the time with focus. Now, every day, take a step toward those goals. Thinking can be a plague. Negativity can be contagious. Think about the rise of Hitler. How did one thought impact the whole world and be responsible for the killing of millions of people? It was contagious. One man stood up and pushed his views onto thousands of other people, and instead of acting on their own beliefs inherent in them as humans, they allowed that negativity to influence their actions. They not only allowed the thought of another person to influence their actions, they allowed the thought of another person to change their minds; their belief of right and wrong.

Negativity is a contagion. When it reaches mass amounts of individuals who are willing to allow it to shape their minds and their actions, such as in pre-World War II Germany, it shows that it can have drastic global effects. Although it is said that Hitler had an incredible ability to persuade and motivate the masses by making them feel as if he were speaking directly to them when speaking to thousands, and he was clearly well versed in exploiting this mental weakness in humanity, without thousands of people allowing him to manipulate their consciousness, he never would have succeeded in any of it.

Do not be a sheep. Do not be afraid to be different. Trust in yourself that you know what is best for you at all times, because really, deep down, you know you do. Everyone does. Everyone, at their core, if they really look deep into themselves in an honest way, knows what they truly want out of life. The only question is, are you brave enough to put yourself out there and get it? Are you willing to do things that are scary, uncomfortable, and uncertain? I know that I was always willing to switch my job in order to have a better gym schedule. That was a key deciding factor in the places I have worked, and that will remain a huge role in where I go in the future. It also determines where I am willing to live.

I don't have a home gym. I have had my own equipment in the past, but I just find that I have more drive when I go to a place that is specifically designed to achieve what I want to achieve. If I have a piece of equipment at home next to a couch, I just don't have the same drive to lift that weight while I look at that comfy couch. There are too many distractions at home, so I personally don't like to mix home with training. The main point is, I don't let those aspects of life affect the goals I want to achieve. Be willing to do what you have to do. Manipulate everything you can, and leave everything else behind. Manipulate your work schedule; use resources like childcare at the gym, afterschool programs if you have kids, meal services, delivery services—anything that helps you to get to where you want to be. Take it one day at a time. If you can keep getting to the gym day in and day out, you get closer and closer to where you want to be. Make sure, if you have a hectic life, to plan ahead. Take one day a week and plan for the rest of the days. Plan your meals, do your grocery shopping, cook, do meal prep, plan your social time and your personal time with significant others. Failing to plan is planning to fail. If you are keeping an eye on your diet and you know you need to eat at 3:00 p.m. but won't be home to cook or around food until seven, make a peanut butter sandwich and put it in your pocket, because come 6:00 p.m., your temptation to eat what you weren't planning on eating will skyrocket. If you know what you are eating and it's ready for you, the chances of you failing that day decrease significantly. If you know you are going to work out the next day, do your laundry and pack your bag the night before so you can just pick it up and go the next day. Be prepared can sometimes make the difference in following through on your plans. Be ready, and try to predict what life is going to throw at you, so when life starts u throwing s**t balls at you, you can knock 'em outta the park.

———

Confucius said "Those who believe they can and those who believe they can't are both often right."

It all starts with faith. You have to have complete faith in your ability to obtain what you are seeking. Most people who rise to incredible heights have come from a place of utter desperation and despair. They have been pushed so low that they see success as their only option left in life. The most incredible acts of change often come from a place of tremendous trauma or severe de-pression. You must have belief in your abilities, belief in your worth, believe that you deserve more than what you have, that you are valuable, that you have more to give than what you are currently expressing to the world. Even if you are at a point right now where you don't believe that, I want you to say out loud to yourself right now: "I believe I am valuable. I believe I have more in me to give. I am worth more than what I am currently expressing to the world. I believe I can create my life as I want it to be."

If you say this (or things like this) to yourself on a daily basis, your subconscious mind will eventually start to believe this and will start moving you in that direction.

The mind is the most remarkable part of the human make-up. Not the brain, the mind. They are separate. The brain is physical; the mind is intangible. The body is not controlled by the brain. It is controlled by the mind. The brain simply allows the mind to bring thoughts into physical manifestation through movement and interaction with the perceived environment. The brain only takes direction from your mind and transfers your desires into your environment. It takes your will and begins to adjust your environment to grant what you are willing. The longer you hold the focus of your mind on your will—or in other words, your desire, your intent, your goal—the more action your body will take toward its fruition.

If you continue doing this without fail, or even with perseverance through failure, it is literally impossible for you not to reach your goal. This goes for any goal or desire you set for yourself. It is important for you to realize that the action portion of this process involves physical effort, in other words *work*! If your goal is to write an essay, your mind will produce it in physical form by having your hand write the words. If this is your desire, your body will make it so. You focus your mind for the amount of time it takes you to write your desired length of essay, and your body will complete it. In the grand scheme of things, the time it takes to focus on writing an essay is minuscule compared to applying focus to your whole life, but it works the same way.

It works the same with shopping for clothing. Your mind says, *I need a new shirt*, and it begins to take action by moving your legs and getting you into the car, driving the car, and walking you into a store to make that purchase. If you lose focus and become distracted by driving instead to another store that sells, let's say beer, and you return home to have a nap instead of continuing to the shirt store, well, it's pretty obvious you won't be reaching the shirt goal you set for yourself that day. Same goes for your appearance. If you focus your mind long enough on the necessary movements you need your body to perform in order to develop the physical features you desire, you will continue to grow in that way. Your dedication to focusing your mind will determine the time required to reach your desired destination.

The more you become distracted from that goal, or the longer your focus is off that goal, the longer it will take to reach. You need to plant that goal in your mind every day and focus on it *every day*. If all your mind consists of is other distraction and mumbo jumbo and isn't focused on your goal, then you can't expect your body to move toward what you really want. You simply can't plant corn and expect potatoes.

If your life currently is in turmoil, your way of thinking is what is causing you the distress. You can't hide from death; we all share this one fate, but changing your thought is how you can be more alive in life. Your life is only yours; you are the one in control, your mind is in the driver's seat, and your body is your vehicle. There are other vehicles and obstacles you may have to overcome, but ultimately, you can choose to maintain your vehicle to the highest standard, so when you need to put the hammer down, it's going to outperform the competition and get you to where you need to be. Look after it, flush its systems, keep tread on the tires, fill it with premium, and don't look in the rear-view mirror when you're leading the pack. Focus on the finish line.

FOCUS

I TRULY BELIEVE this world is full of people who are incredibly talented in all areas of life, but they fail to use their minds and bodies in unison to focus on what they want and take appropriate action in a timely manner to manifest their true potential into the world. They either fail to find and develop what would most fulfill them, or they become distracted in their attempts at its manifestation. Motivation is really unreliable in the sense that it really only sparks your interest. The human mind *never* feels like doing anything uncomfortable. It is up to you to force your mind into discomfort and strain. The mind *always* wants you to maintain comfort. But growth simply does not come from being comfortable; it comes from discomfort and pain. It comes from being forced into discomfort and fighting to get that comfort back. This is where the old saying, "no pain, no gain" comes from. In order to know comfort, you must know discomfort. In order to know success, you must know failure. The mind always wants you to be comfortable; it is designed to seek comfort and homeostasis for your body.

Think of running, for example. Every second, your mind is telling you to stop. Your will and desire are what you are using to fight against your physical body and your mind telling you to stop if is no danger is present. Your body wants to conserve that energy for times when you are in danger, in order to incite the fight-or-flight response along with the adrenaline release. The time you are able to sustain your physical movement beyond what your body considers comfortable is completely proportionate to the strength of your will and desire to continue the action against your body's outcry. You just need to decide what you want. Make a decision. Just decide on it. If you want to make change, make a decision and commit to it. Do not decide to try. Decide and commit to success 100 percent. Cut off all other outcomes, and decide on change and nothing else. Every second you spend being afraid to make a decision is time you will never get back toward your goal.

There are billions of people on Earth who are trying to do the same thing. Succeed. If you decide and commit, you are instantly in the leading percentile. Strive with dedication and commitment through failure and through frustration. If you reach a sticking point, think for a moment about why these obstacles appeared, devise a plan to fix it, accept the setback, and continue pushing forward. Failure is not the point where you reach a setback or a loss. Failure really happens when you decide to no longer pick yourself back up and continue striving for the end product. Treat failure as success in learning more about yourself in the process. Question what thinking led you into that predicament and what can you change in order to limit the possibility of reaching this point again or how to work on overcoming it faster next time.

Paths to success never come in the form of a well-groomed walking trail. They are often a mixture of formed sidewalk, marshlands, and the Himalayan Mountains. The best you can do is expect the worst and pack accordingly. Your limitations set by the mind are the terrain, and your positive thoughts and focus are your survival equipment. Failure can be the most powerful aspect of your journey; it is how you interpret it that makes all the difference. You can choose to allow the failure to stop you from proceeding and not get what you want, or you can be one of the people who succeed at getting what they want out of life. Few people get what they want; the majority, do not. Which person do you want to be? It is a decision; it's not a fate. You can have anything you want in life, but you have to be willing to put in the work. You have to match your discipline and effort with what you want. If you aren't willing to do that, you can't expect to make it to your destination.

Just start. It is very inconvenient. It will never *be* convenient. You have to realize that. But every person who has ever done anything worthy of great praise goes through these tremendous difficulties. If you are unwilling to go through these hardships, do not complain about your situation. Do not make excuses. When you make excuses, all you are doing is telling others about your character flaws. You are pointing out where you are weak. And really, no one gives a s**t. No one wants to hear why you couldn't do something. If you are trying to get somewhere or get something, your excuses aren't going to get you there. Realize your weaknesses. They are steps in your staircase on the way up. They may be cracked, broken, and unsteady, but you still need to get past them in order to keep climbing. Realize them, know them intimately, and conquer them as micro-successes toward your greater goal.

These small successes, the overcoming of your weaknesses along the way, will turn you into the person who can conquer your ultimate goal. Overcoming your weaknesses is fundamental to developing your character. The faster you can observe these weaknesses as an uninvolved observer of your behavior and make the appropriate changes to your behavior and your thinking, the faster you can move on to the next step. The more you do this, the more you overcome, the faster you get at this process. You become extremely efficient at identifying the issues and making choices, to the point where it becomes automatic. Again, you have to be willing to honestly observe your behavior and your thoughts as a third party, be honest with yourself, and see your weakness. Admit them to yourself. You must be honest with yourself. *Yeah, I really suck at this. Yeah, I really made a bad choice there. I have a weakness choosing correctly in that area*, and so on.

You must realize your flaws and work on them. When you make excuses for your flaws, you are making an argument for your stagnation. You are pleading a case, trying to justify why you should accept the failure you have come across. Your mind is convincing your body to remain comfortable in your current state and not take the steps to exit that comfort zone and conquer all that stands in your way. Even people who are serious, seasoned weightlifters sometimes fall into these psychological traps. Power lifting is a completely different activity than what I practice and there are many people competing in that sport who don't care about aesthetics. However, in my opinion, a large number of those who are powerlifters choose their path because of the lack of responsibility needed in caloric and macro restriction. A lot of the people who fall into this category love being strong and lifting heavy weights but lack the discipline or will to cut their body fat down, which is a shame because some of the most insane examples of the superhuman physiques have come from powerlifting-style dominant routines mixed with bodybuilding-style dieting regimens.

Take Ronnie Colman or Branch Warren, for example. They are quite interesting people. Mind you, performance enhancement plays a role in those cases, but they are examples of incredible physiques built with elements of powerlifting and calorie/nutrient manipulation. A lot of these people who just lack the discipline will tell you they don't want to be aesthetic. From the people I have spoken to who fall into this category, it is my opinion that it is easier to make those excuses and pretend you want a physique that comes from not having the discipline to restrict your diet than to accept that fact that you are lying to yourself and develop the mental toughness needed to do something about it. Put it this way: if there were a physique department store, the man boobs would be on permanent clearance.

NO EXCUSES – LOSE YOUR EGO

THE ONLY WAY to get what you want is to recognize this and move to get your desired results. No one cares about why you can't do something. The only thing people care about is the outcome. If you are working a job and want a promotion, your boss does not care about why you couldn't get something done. The only thing he cares about are the results. The promotion will always go to the guy who has the results. So, the faster you overcome these flaws that are holding you back, the faster you get results, the faster you will climb to your goal. Do not be concerned with others. Do not compare your path to others'. It does not make a difference if your path is easier or harder than someone else's. You still need to get over your own hurdles. You can't use the excuse, "Oh, he has the time," or "He has the money," or "It's easy for them because of such and such." No! Everyone who succeeds in his or her personal goals goes through struggle. Theirs may be different than yours, but anyone who has the desire to accomplish substantial personal success and bring those ideas into the world *must* go through the same process.

Yes, if you have more money, resources may be more readily available in some aspects, but such people still have to do battle within themselves to strive, to create, to form ideas, to plan, to hustle, to have discipline, and simply to *get up and get s**t done.* If you can't make yourself do the things you need to do, you will never get where you want to be. Comparing yourself to others only takes time away from working toward your end result. Your *ego* will end your progress if you let it. Inside the gym or outside in life, your ego will control your gains if you let it. If you are walking into the gym and throwing on as much weight as you can, banging out half repetitions to look and feel bigger than you are, you are *losing.* If you are sitting on the bench press or squat rack with 315 pounds loaded up, waiting for people to care and take notice, you are losing.

The people who are winning aren't looking at you and applauding. If they know what they are doing, they are laughing to themselves and pulling ahead in the race. They know that you are far behind psychologically, and until you make a change mentally, you will never get on their level. The same goes for life. If you are buying that seventy-thousand-dollar vehicle to feel larger than you are but earn forty thousand dollars a year, you are in the same situation. You have not yet reached the point where you can properly own that item and live comfortably. You simply have not yet earned that life-style. You are trying to appear as something you are not, in order to be applauded by others, without having to put the work in. All the while, you're spending energy, ignoring that thought that sits in the back of your mind, reminding you, letting you know you haven't really earned the ability you are portraying. You are not really that person you are trying to be.

The longer you keep pretending and lying to yourself, the longer you will stay in that situation. There are no short cuts to success. Go to the gym and do your reps with the appropriate weight, and when you have put in the work, your body will move you up to the next level. The CEO of the company usually never starts a career off in that position. He or she may have to get an internship in the mailroom first. Life does the same thing, but you have to be willing to build the equity first. Hustle your ass off. Drive that rusty beast into the ground while you are building, and life will reward you. If you are always too worried about what other people are doing, you will do nothing but waste time focused on them that could be spent climbing higher. You must master your mind. Realize when it is holding you back, and take control of it. Treat it like that rusty beast you're flying down the road. Keep a firm grip on that steering wheel, and pin the throttle. Never stop trying to progress in your thinking. Never take your hands off the wheel. Your mind has unlimited potential. Your limits are only what you believe them to be. If you keep working on your thought process and overcoming hurdle after hurdle, there are no limits to your potential. You can overcome anything!

It all starts in the mind. Take charge of your thoughts. Do not partake in the negative self-talk that your mind will push on you. That is your mind keeping you comfortable. When you realize your mind is pushing negativity and doubt on you, it's up to you to force thoughts of success and positive self-talk and positive affirmation onto it. Replace *I am not* with *I am*. Replace *I can't* with *I can*. Even if at first you don't believe them, the more you tell yourself *I can* or *I am*, the more you are hypnotizing your subconscious mind to accept that truth. Instead of *I'm not smart enough*, state in your mind *I am incredibly intelligent*. Instead of *I can't*, state *I can do anything I want if I want it badly enough. I can create whatever I want to create in life*. When you believe you are capable of success, you automatically become **successful** in believing it is possible. You have already begun to succeed. That is your first hurdle. Now keep running.

The majority of people never take this control of their minds. If you want to reach heights most other people never reach, you have to think differently than most other people think. Just get started. The clock is ticking. You can always make more money, but you can't make time. You don't have to start off as a success to become successful. But you have to start. Make a plan and begin to take action at once. What knowledge do you need? Go get it. What services do you require? Go find them. What resources are available? Use them. What talent do you have? What are you good at? What fulfills you? What are you passionate about? Whatever it is, just get going, because life is too short to sit around telling stories about why you didn't do what you really know you should have done.

I know I don't want to be on my deathbed, regretting all the hopes and dreams I never even attempted. I want to know that I gave everything I had. I used all my talent to its greatest potential and did not use excuses to hide from my shortcomings. Think about what success is to you, and that is your end goal. Fight for it. Fight for it like you have nothing left to lose. One thing I learned working in the prison system is that the most dangerous people are the ones who fight with nothing left to lose. Fight like you have nothing left to lose. Be dangerous. No one else cares about your goal. No one is going to achieve it for you, and no one is going to believe in it for you. We all have greatness inside of us. You need to be courageous enough to take that challenge in bringing it out of your mind and into the physical world. Let the world see the potential within you. Don't shy away from showing others what you are capable of, and don't allow the opinions of others to affect your progress. Show them what you are worth, and you will be compensated for it. It all starts with your thinking. It begins with the belief in yourself and the belief in the limitless possibilities that your mind can create.

> If you can see it in your mind,
> you can hold it in your hand.
> —Bob Proctor

Some of your hardest battles are going to be fought against the people you are closest with. Romantic relationships are the hardest ones. Your biggest critic may just be the person you share your entire life with. You may be with someone who just does not realize what your goals mean to you and has no interest in supporting them. You cannot fold to this person, though. You cannot live for what he or she wants. You absolutely need to live for yourself. Do not live for others. If you live for the negative opinion of your romantic partner, you could find yourself one day looking back at the time you spent not working on what you wanted to achieve, not accomplishing your goals, and regret that now you are short on time. I know that I personally could not be OK with that. I know that fundamentally I cannot be happy if I am not personally progressing in what I consider to be a worthy ideal. Your partner may never understand why you need to do what you are doing or understand the satisfaction it brings you. This person doesn't realize the importance those goals play in your overall development of yourself as a person and sees you spending time at the gym as time that you should be spending with him or her instead—unable to see what you believe in. The irony in this situation is a lot of people are motivated to better themselves in order to be a better person for the one they love, but it can be that same person who slows their progress.

There is also the possibility that, like other people you will come across, you bettering yourself in areas may make your partner feel inferior and feel like making improvements in those same areas, even though those things aren't important to his or her own journey. If it's fitness, people may feel insecure if they are not in great shape themselves, and they see you beginning to achieve success in that area. If this is the case, it is important to talk with them about it and let them know that you are not doing this to compete with anyone but yourself. It has nothing to do with how anyone else looks. It has to do with how you feel. *I feel good when I work on my goals.*

Let your partner know that he or she is on his or her own path and you love him or her for the person he or she is. Provide information on what you are doing and why you want to do it. It's not about anyone else; it's about your personal goals and reaching others. If your partner is the type who always gives you grief about going to the gym, this is where you need to take a serious stand. This will really show you what you want and test how badly you want it. You have to be prepared to *be selfish!* You have to stand up for how you want to live your life and not let anyone, *anyone*, not even the woman or man of your dreams, the one you love more than anyone else (other than yourself) tell you not to work on what is important to you in your life. You have to be willing to walk out that door and allow the other person to stew; go do your routine, and forget about what anyone else thinks. This will not only test how badly you want it but will test how strong your relationship is and how much the person you are with really loves and supports you. You have to risk the turmoil. You have to be willing to break him or her in like a wild horse. Eventually, your partner will either run away or be tamed.

SACRIFICE

Overall, you are going to have to be willing to make sacrifices. If you are a very social person, this could be a difficult hurdle for you. If you are out socializing most days or nights of the week and that is part of who you are, you are going to have to make some serious changes that may involve limiting and prioritizing certain relationships. You may need to sit down and think about them and find out the ones that are taking time away from reaching your goals or are negatively influencing your behavior and throwing you off your mindset. The younger you are, the more difficult this can be. Most younger people are not yet fully developed into who they are comfortable being, which should be themselves. When you are younger, you are still highly influenced by the opinions of others, because you don't yet have complete confidence in who you are or who you want to become. This can make it very hard to say no when asked to partake in social functions like parties or trips to the bar.

You have to be willing to risk relationships that may not be completely vital to you, like those of work colleagues or acquaintances. If you know you are going to be too tempted not to adhere to your dietary needs or are going to be pressured to consume large amounts of alcohol, you will need to make the sacrifice of not going out that night in order to meet your goals. Yes, this is part of it. Not getting everything you want and limiting instant gratification through self-restraint is paramount in your success. The more you practice having control of your mind, using it to dominate your body, and making yourself do what you know you need to succeed, the better and more efficient you will be. If you do choose to socialize, you have to be willing to be "that guy" (or girl) who drinks water all night or who orders the salad with dressing on the side *and own that role!* People may make fun of you and criticize you, perhaps making comments like "Live a little" and "You only live once." That's right. You only live once, so do it your way, not theirs.

When you are on your deathbed someday, are you going to look back and think about that pound of chicken wings that night or that pint of beer you didn't drink? No. You are going to think about whether you reached your goals and dreams and whether or not you accomplished what you desired your life to be. No one reaches goals and realizes dreams by living a life of gluttony and not utilizing self-control. You have to be able to see your future, believe it is possible, and continue pushing toward it. The more you avoid straying off your path, however hard it may be, the further into the distance the easy road fades, until there is only one option—success.

ALCOHOL BAD, CANNABIS GOOD (MAYBE...)

ALCOHOL AND FITNESS don't mix for reasons anyone can easily understand. Alcohol has hundreds of negative effects on your body. These negative effects include harming the stomach, pancreas, skin, kidneys, and bones, as well as sexual health and fertility. Alcohol negatively affects the heart, lungs, brain, and the overall mental health of the user. Alcohol is a depressant. It is full of sugar, throws your body into unhealthy chaos, and makes you feel awful. As with any aspect of life, moderation is key. If you are out at the bar multiple times per week, it shouldn't be a mystery to you why you aren't reaching your goals. Alcohol has been shown to slow the protein synthesis in the body. Consuming alcohol produces harmful byproducts in the body, and it limits the body's ability to absorb nutrients efficiently.

Studies have shown that even moderate alcohol consumption can decrease your testosterone levels. However, other studies show that a small amount of alcohol—meaning one drink per day, as in one serving, 250 ml or one cup, not one drink the size of a bucket—has positive effects on the vascular system and heart function. Personally, I abstain from alcohol most of the time because of its caloric content alone. Not only that, but I really hate the way excessive alcohol consumption makes me feel. It just slows me down. It brings any progress I am making in life, in any area, to a grinding halt. It's not that I don't live life up at times; I am just very selective of the times I indulge in that side of things. I still consume a glass of red wine some nights during the week, or on the weekend have a couple pints of beer, but for me to get that third sheet catching the wind, there had better be a serious occasion happening like a wedding, a New Year's Eve party, or a sunny vacation somewhere. You still need to celebrate life at times and enjoy it to the fullest, but you don't need to celebrate that it's Tuesday night and you bought some socks.

The use of cannabis, however, is a lot more contested. I myself have arguments for the use of cannabis, as well as arguments against it. But anything you consume or partake in that causes detriment, stagnation, or regression in regards to your goals or your life in general, you should most definitely abstain. That being said, it is again a matter of moderation and responsible use. It doesn't take a scientist to resolve that inhaling burning pieces of plant matter into your lungs is not the best thing you could be doing for your respiratory system. However, there are many ways to consume the cannabis plant that involves eliminating the smoke by-products from burning the plant in order to reap the benefits it can provide. If the use of cannabis results in you not accomplishing your goals, sleeping too long, eating too much of what you shouldn't be eating, not working out, not going to school, or issues in your relationships, then you should 100 percent abstain from it. Every person is different in how they respond to the effects of cannabis. Some people just cannot mentally handle the cognitive stimulation it provides, while in others, it can cause intense impulses of creativity, clarity of thought, and reason beyond what they are used to experiencing under normal conditions. It can cause a lack of motivation but can also cause some people to have an incredible amount. It can cause an uplifted energetic and euphoric sense of drive and passion but can also induce anxiety and depression. It is completely up to the user's mental health, intellectual capacity, and history of use, as well as the potency, chemical makeup of the strain of plant being utilized, and the environment and state of mind the user is in a time of consumption.

There are many varying factors that could either benefit or be of detriment to the user. It is no secret now as Western countries move toward legalization of cannabis (Canada is set for July 2018) that cannabis has been shown to have an array of positive effects on the mind and the body. The most beneficial to the person partaking in fitness training would be the assistance it can provide in getting a good night's rest and the anti-inflammatory and muscle-relaxation properties it contains. I personally have used cannabis quite a bit in the past, although now I only utilize it every so often as a way to help moderate and maintain my mental health. After hustling at life for extended periods, I want to ensure a solid night of rest. To be completely honest, I have had incredible leaps and bounds in the understanding of how my body moves and works in the weight room by experimenting with cannabis and bodybuilding for some of my years in the gym. I have found, only through my own personal experimentation in my younger years, that cannabis allowed me not only to be able to push my body to its limits through increasing my very will to succeed; it allowed me to make the most intense mind-muscle connections while lifting, to be able to achieve the exact angles I needed my limbs to find in order to zero in on the muscle group I was aiming to exhaust.

I found this aspect of cannabis use to be the most beneficial and the most helpful of any supplement, dietary aid, or workout style I have ever tried. The connection you have with your body in the weight room while under the influence of cannabis is an incredible feeling. I feel as though I have never had a deeper understanding of how my mind and my physical body work in unison and how my mind is in complete control of what is possible. It can also be very useful for meditation, self-reflection, and setting priorities and goals.

> "When you smoke the herb,
> it reveals you to yourself."
> —Bob Marley

> "The body is very important, but the mind is
> more important than the body."
> —Arnold Schwarzenegger

That second quote, by the way, as simple as it may be, is by someone who also utilized cannabis while achieving his goals in the weight room. He won seven Mr. Olympia competitions. He then became a Hollywood blockbuster movie star and the governor of California. Just keep that in mind. Do I recommend individuals use cannabis? No. Do I recommend they use cannabis and go lift weights over their heads? No. But you are your own person, and I am only telling you my own experiences. I recommend you do research on the subject and make your own conclusions. That is what this is about. I am sharing with you how I have succeeded in my goals. This is one aspect that has helped me significantly. What you choose to do is up to you.

No one influenced me to make these choices; I chose for myself as a free-thinking adult. If you have no experience with the effects of cannabis, would common sense tell you to go get intoxicated and lift weights over your head? No. But if you are a seasoned lifter and you have a great deal of experience with both weight training and cannabis use, you may one day choose to blend the two together and take your workouts to outer space. That's your choice. Keep in mind that substance dependency is ultimately a form of weakness and will become a detriment whether it is preworkout, sugar, or cannabis. The bottom line is, if you find that the use is beneficial to you, then keep on keeping on. But be honest with yourself. If you find that it is holding you back, even a little bit, from reaching that next level you want to get to, it may be time to rethink your priorities and turn off the Bob Marley.

———

UTILIZING THE LAW OF ATTRACTION

THE LAW OF attraction is an understood law of the intangible universe that consists of your own thoughts creating your reality. In short, we become what we think about. The modern idea of this law was brought on by the book *The Secret* by Rhonda Byrne, published in 2006 and made very popular when featured on *The Oprah Winfrey Show*. The book has sold over twenty million copies worldwide and has been translated into fifty different languages. However, this book was influenced by other books speaking of this thinking method, with modern publications dating back to 1910. The book *The Edinburgh Lectures on Mental Science* (1904), by English author Thomas Troward is one example. Other authors who are considered to be part of this so called new thought movement are Wallace D. Wattles, who authored the book *The Science of Getting Rich*, James Allen, who wrote *As a Man Thinketh*, and Napoleon Hill, who wrote *Think and Grow Rich*. These books all contain the same basic principles of thought. Though they date back to the mid-nineteenth century, if you study the history of man, these same principles of thought have been noted and practiced by the greatest minds that have ever existed in human history. The common message is that when you control your thoughts, you control your life. Point your thoughts toward what you want, maintain focus on that, work steadily toward it, and you must succeed.

> All that we are is the result of what we have thought. The mind is everything. What we think we become.
> —Buddha

> Everything is energy and that's all there is to it. Match the frequency of the reality you want and you cannot help but get that reality. It can be no other way. This is not philosophy. This is physics.
> —Albert Einstein

> Imagination is everything. It is the preview of life's coming attractions.
> —Albert Einstein

Be careful about what you think. Your thoughts
run your life.
—Jesus Christ

Everything is possible for he who believes.
—Mark 9:23

If you focus your thoughts daily on accomplishing a goal you genuinely feel is possible and you take action, working steadily toward this goal, you will reach it. This is the basic teaching. The reason I am including this section is because I realized I was using this thinking method *after* practicing what it preaches. I utilized this method of focusing my thoughts every day, as often as possible. I would visualize what I wanted to look like and visualize myself going through the process—in the gym, eating meals, what clothes I would wear, how I would feel. I created collages on my computer to use as my desktop, I watched motivational videos every day, I listened to motivational speeches and watched motivational movies like *Rocky* and *The Pursuit of Happyness* as often as possible. My whole life, every spare second that wasn't spent on other obligations was spent thinking and acting toward reaching my goal of becoming lean enough to see my abs.

I had no idea what the law of attraction was until a friend suggested I read a book called *A Happy Pocket*

Full of Money, written by David Cameron Gikandi. This book opened my eyes to what I was doing. Without even knowing it, I was utilizing a thought process that many other very successful people had been practicing for centuries. I went on YouTube, and when I searched "Law of Attraction," I came across celebrities talking about how they reached such heights only by way of changing the way they were thinking. It was amazing and a huge turning point in my life to see and hear so many successful people crediting their success to thinking the way I had been thinking—celebrities such as Arnold Schwarzenegger, Will Smith, Steve Harvey, Denzel Washington, Jim Carrey, Jay-Z, Tyler Perry, Lady Gaga, LMFAO, UFC fighters Connor McGregor and Jon Jones, Richard Gere, Eva Mendez, and Pierce Brosnan, just to name a few. All these people were talking about the same method of thought that they attribute to their success. It was mind-blowing. I was so intrigued that there was so much information on this way of thinking that out of pure curiosity, I began reading the suggested works these people were mentioning that had helped them, and I suggest that you do the same. If nothing else, these books will put you in a positive state of mind and help you in times when you are full of self-doubt or caught in a web of negativity.

So what you have in your life right now is a result of your thinking. If you are always thinking "I'm weak; I'll never make it" or "I'm never going to be successful" or "I'll never be wealthy," you are attracting those things into your life as well. It works both negatively and positively. What you are thinking, you are attracting into your life. A trick I use is to state the opposite of what negative thoughts I am having. When I catch myself thinking negative thoughts like "People drive like assholes," I will state to myself something that contradicts that statement like "I am grateful to own my own vehicle" or "I am grateful I don't have to take the bus" or "I am grateful that I have climate control and music to listen to." I try now to realize when I am having negative thoughts and replace those thoughts with gratitude for the good things I am lucky to have. I have found this to be very helpful in maintaining a positive outlook and maintaining positive focus on the future.

> I would visualize having directors interested in me, people I respected saying "I like your work." I would visualize things coming to me that I wanted. I had nothing at that time, but it just made me feel better. I would drive home and think, *I do have these things. They're out there. I just don't have a hold of them yet, but they're out there.* I wrote myself a check for ten million dollars, for acting services rendered. I dated it Thanksgiving 1995, and I gave myself five years

or three years maybe, and I kept it in my pocket,
and it deteriorated and deteriorated, but then
just before Thanksgiving 1995, I found out I
was gonna make ten million dollars on, I think
it was *Dumb and Dumber*. What we really want
seems impossibly out of reach and ridiculous
to expect, so we never dare to ask the universe
for it. I'm saying I'm the proof. You can ask the
universe for it.
—Jim Carrey

This "law" of attraction that everyone is talking about is not simply an ideology. The reason it is considered by most physicists to be a law of the universe like gravity is, is because it is actually being proven by modern science. For example, I strongly encourage you to research the "double slit experiment." Versions of this experiment date back to the nineteenth century, when scientists were studying the properties of light waves. The latest versions of the experiment by Dr. Richard Feynman conclude that the simple fact that there is an observer in place affects the way atoms behave. Simply put, the subatomic particles of energy are effected by an observer being present. When no observer is present they respond in a different manner. This question could be asked, are the particles are somehow *aware*, they are being observed? Science is still trying to comprehend this phenomenon in its entirety. Subatomic particles are basically tiny balls of energy. They do not make energy. They *are* energy. They are the source of all creation in the universe. They are the fabric of our reality, and science is proving that they have their own awareness. There is a great video on YouTube that explains this to the layman. Search for Professor Jim Al-Khalili, Central Mystery of Quantum Mechanics, and the double slit experiment.

Another experiment that is very intriguing is the Water Experiment by Dr. Masaru Emoto. This is an experiment where Dr. Emoto took water samples, froze them, and studied the crystals under a microscope. Water crystals take on the same sort of form as a snowflake does. They are all different. His initial research was to note the difference in the ice crystals from different water sources. What Dr. Emoto actually discovered was that the most beautiful crystals formed when he was playing beautiful music. What is the significance of this? It suggests that indeed, everything is energy and everything feels energy. We are all connected. The water can feel the music. It is aware, somehow, of the waves of sound energy and its frequency being transmitted. That energy is being felt and absorbed by the water and is shaping its existence.

How does this pertain to our state of mind, our lives, and our goals? Consider that music is vibrational energy, just like our thoughts and our words; our bodies are made up of about 72 percent water. The vibrations of energy in life we expose ourselves to affect our bodies on a molecular level. If you expose yourself to dark, negative, and dysfunctional situations and people, you are affecting the very make-up of your being. That energy is absorbed by your body, and it will have a negative impact on your mind and the vibrational energy that you yourself give off. Dr. Emoto also believes that our thoughts create our reality, and if that is true, the impact that negativity has on our minds will hinder the creation of our optimal reality. So be careful what you allow into your life. It could be what holds you back from achieving your desires.

I became aware of this experiment in my younger years through a DVD I watched called *What the Bleep! Down the Rabbit Hole*, a documentary on quantum mechanics and neurobiology that includes interviews with quantum theorists and scientists from around the world, including Fred Alan Wolf, Daniel Monti, Stuart Hameroff, and John Hagelin. I became interested in learning about quantum mechanics from reading Stephen Hawking's book *The Theory of Everything*, published in 2002, in which Hawking speaks about important theories involving time and space. He also talks about many of the most complex theories from modern physics in a way that even people with a substantially lower IQ, like myself, can comprehend. I would recommend it for developing a greater understanding of the way our universe operates and how much mystery still exists in our daily lives that goes unconsidered by the majority of our society by being intangible and, to most, incomprehensible. When you expand your mind, you will expand the limits of your body. If you are able to push your thinking to its limits, you will be more capable of pushing your body as well. In order to grow, you need to grow in all areas of your existence. It is impossible to achieve physical growth without the simultaneous growth of your state of mind.

> I'll do whatever it takes. The number of hours
> it takes. The visualization. Looking at train-
> ing footage. Looking at motivational books.
> Reading this. Reading that. Whatever it takes I
> will do. And that hunger you have to develop,
> because you have to create a goal for yourself,
> whatever that may be. A short-term goal and a
> long-term goal and you got to go after that. And
> if you do not see it and you do not believe it,
> who else will? So now you apply that principle to
> acting. Let's go to acting class every day. Let's go
> and work on the accent with the same amount
> of time. With the same amount of will. Let's

visualize it: What am I shooting for? I want to be another Clint Eastwood, I want to be another John Wayne, Kirk Douglas, all of these great heroes I admired as a kid. So that's what I'm going after. And that same principle works. Even though there are so many people around that say no, you will never make it because you have an accent, you know, your body is too big and your name Schwarzen Schnitzel or whatever. Doesn't matter if anyone else knows or if anyone else believes in it. *You* know. And that *you* know that principle, visualizing yourself as a star will work and all you have to do now is go toward that vision. And really that's what I always believed in, and I feel like that is the only way you can get ahead. If you have a very clear vision where you want to go and if you are willing to put the work in, no matter what it takes to get them to turn this vision into reality. We can accomplish basically anything you want.
—Arnold Schwarzenegger

When I first started weight training, I used to hold the belief that only people with certain body types could ever reach the goal of having six-pack abs. Then one day, after thinking to myself for a long period of time, I made a decision: I was going to do it. I didn't know how yet, but this was something I had always dreamed of obtaining, and I realized that I was just lying to myself, making excuses why I couldn't do it. I believed I could not obtain what I wanted, without even putting in the work and effort needed to even give it opportunity to manifest. I just *decided* to do it and not let anything stand in my way. To do what was necessary and commit to success. So what did I do? I started researching. I read, I educated myself on what diets and nutrition I would need to be familiar with; nutrition, meal timing, workout styles, what those who had reached my goal utilized and had success with. I downloaded pictures of what I wanted to look like. I watched endless YouTube videos of people who had reached my goal, and I plucked relevant information from an incredible amount of resources. I tried what others had success in trying; I watched motivational videos, I read motivational books, and I talked to people at the gym and asked questions.

Everything I did for a year and a half involved working toward that goal. All my spare time was focused on that. I listened to motivational speeches while I slept. I worked out five, six, sometimes seven days a week. I adhered to a strict diet, and sometimes I would fail and mess up and give in to cravings, but when I failed, I only took that as knowledge I gained about myself and figured out ways to avoid falling back into that same situation. I didn't just give up at the first failure. I failed many times and kept getting back on the horse. I accepted that failure is part of the journey, and if you fail enough and recover enough, you eventually get better at the recovery. The recovery becomes habit in itself. Soon, the period of time between failing and recovery becomes smaller and smaller. Like anything, the more you fail, the better you get at it. This is how badly I wanted it, and eventually after many failed attempts and many recoveries, I reached my goal, a goal that I once firmly believed was impossible—*impossible.*

I believed that never in my life I would be able to achieve what I achieved. But I forced myself to believe. I brainwashed myself with positive affirmation and focus, visual and audio stimuli and daily self-coaching into believing it was possible. I said to myself, "I am able; it is possible," over and over daily and visualizing what I wanted to look like over and over while taking action, developing a disciplined personality, not caring about other people's opinions, and putting in the hard work. I succeeded in what I once thought impossible. So then I began to think: What are the other beliefs I hold to be impossible? If I could manipulate one area of my mind to bring what I believed impossible into existence, then why couldn't I utilize this same process for other areas? After this experience, my mind was never the same again. My thought process had completely changed, and

I began to tear down the negative and limiting beliefs I had about myself and life in general.

I believe I can create whatever it is I want to create. There is a flow of the universe. I have grown to know just how to go with it. The first step is you have to believe it. Being realistic is the most commonly traveled road to mediocrity. There is a redemptive power that making a choice has, you know. Rather than feeling like you're at effect to all the things that are happening. Make a choice, right. You just decide. What it's gonna be, who you're gonna be, how you're gonna do it. Just decide. And then from that point, the universe is gonna get out your way.
—Will Smith

CONFIDENCE

THINK OF THAT feeling you get when you buy a brand-new outfit or a suit or a whole new wardrobe. You feel like a million bucks, and it changes the entire way you feel and carry yourself. Now imagine if that new outfit was your own skin. Imagine the confidence you would feel. The sheer fact that you have to cover some of it up would come across as a damn shame to you. That is what reaching your aesthetic goals can do for you. Not only will you feel incredible, but you will give off the vibrational energy that will attract people and opportunity to you. People will want to be near you. People will want to know you. People will want to be you, as well as want to be near you. You will subconsciously be giving off external signals that you have complete faith in your own abilities to do anything you put your mind to. Confidence goes way beyond words. Many people trash talk and boast, but when you are truly confident, you don't need to say much, and sometimes nothing at all. People just *know* you are a boss, and it will make them think twice before fucking with you in any way, shape, or form. You have proven to yourself that you can conquer yourself, your flaws, and commit to becoming the best version of yourself you can be. It shows in your physique and in your body language. You no longer hide behind a plethora of excuses as to why you are mediocre in multiple facets of life. You no longer have anything to hide, since you no longer care about what other people think. In order to get to that level of confidence, you have to let outside influence go and have faith in yourself and your abilities. Have faith that you alone and your beliefs will carry you where you want to be. That scares a lot of people, because some will not actually understand the mind-set you have had to put yourself in. They will simply not be able to comprehend how you have done what you have done and how you have developed the confidence you have. It doesn't just come from how you look. It comes from what you had to overcome mentally to get the physique you have. Others have not come anywhere close to reaching that or even attempting it.

That's why a lot of people will ask you if you are on steroids. To them, there must be some sort of advantage you have over them. Although these same people, when asked how often they work out, can't tell you specifically. When asked how many calories they ate today, they can't answer anywhere close to accurately. When asked for their macronutrient ratios, they don't even know what that means. That is how far removed they are from where you have risen to. By reaching your aesthetic goals, you will be elevating yourself to a level far above 95 percent of society, both physically and mentally. You may not be there yet. You may just be learning about how to get there, but trust me, the journey will change who you are as a person when you reach the destination.

Stop living your life based on other people's opinions of you and start living it based on your own values. Ask yourself if you are living up to your expectations, and don't spend any more time considering if anyone else's are being met. Value your own opinions, regardless of what anyone else thinks. The more you do this, the more you will grow your confidence in yourself. Don't be afraid to live life on your own terms, without regard for anyone else's approval. This does not mean you have the right to be a jerk and to hurt other people's feelings or put others down or act like you are somehow superior to them because you have reached a certain goal.

You still reap what you sow, and if you are a jerk to people who are still working through their own mind and world of problems in order to be happy, that will come back on you later. Instead, it is your responsibility to help others. Help them become who they want to become. Inspire and encourage people. Tell them how you changed your thinking to benefit your life. Don't just say "I work out a lot." Go more in depth. Some people won't want to hear what it actually takes to do what you have done, but you can still try. You will, every once in a while, encounter someone who takes great interest in what you have to say about how you reached your goals. By being encouraging and genuine with people, you could actually set them on their way to a better life, just as something sparked you to begin yours. You never know whose life you can change just by being kind, honest, and genuine.

By being open, genuine, and honest, people will be even more attracted to you, since they can trust you, knowing that what you say you mean, and you have tried to direct them in the best direction possible. When you are presenting the best side of yourself to other people, the only people who will not want to be around you are the people who will see those flaws you are not presenting in themselves and want to ignore them. Therefore, they won't want to be around you, since you remind them of their shortcomings, and they are not yet willing to be honest with themselves.

Many people will look at you with envy and will hate on you just for living life on your terms, since they want to embody those character traits but have not yet had the courage to start developing themselves into that person. There are also people who just don't like you, period, and that's just a fact of life. Don't get those people confused. You will find that those people who don't like you because your successes will attract other people of the same mind-set. They are full of confused admiration, and misery loves company. Those people have a lower state of consciousness than those who are curious about how you have developed into a different person. Those people see the value in speaking with you and getting to know the path you have taken. They have an elevated state of mind that allows them to see the potential a conversation or time spent with you could have to influence their own lives. These are the same people who have the most potential to make those changes in themselves, as they are on an elevated plane already above the confused admirers.

Always be humble and grateful, even when being hated by others. Be thankful that you have the ability to withstand the negativity other people project because of the realization of their inadequacies, and be grateful that you have had the mental fortitude to overcome what they are battling within themselves. Don't forget as well that there are people out there who know more than you. There always will be, so never mistake constructive criticism for hate. Always have that in the back of your mind, and don't just dismiss everything that people who may know what they are talking about are saying to you, if it sounds like it may help you or make you a stronger person.

If you have complete confidence in what you are doing, keep going. You will always encounter criticism if you are trying to do anything different; it can't be avoided. There are billions of people in the world, and every single one of them has an opinion. Aristotle said, "If you don't want to be criticized, say nothing, do nothing, be nothing." If you do anything different than the majority are doing, you will definitely be criticized. One of the fastest roads to mediocrity is spending time trying to please everyone. Spend as little time as possible around those who carry negativity, and spend as much time as you can with those who embody the spirit you believe in. Ultimately, the confidence you develop will not only make you feel incredible; it will develop your mind to the point where dealing with negativity becomes as easy as brushing off your shoulder.

Part of confidence is the courage to be yourself. So many people are striving to appear as something they are not. They are trying to be larger than life while out at the club and trying to appear stronger than they are at the gym. Having the courage to be yourself is a big part of success in the gym. You can't fake results there. You have either reached your goal or you haven't, and it's always on display for everyone to see. Whether you are walking into a boardroom or walking into the gym, straighten your back, retract your shoulders, hold your head high, be proud of who you are, and don't be afraid to show that person to the world.

Unfortunately, there is no quick fix when it comes to bodybuilding, muscle development, and fat loss. In reality, it takes many *years* of consistency to achieve the physique most people would consider their ideal or dream body composition, with diet and nutrition being a higher priority than weight training. Many individuals are in love with the idea of having an incredible physique but do not understand that it is not a hobby or a pastime; this is a lifestyle. If you want to achieve the ultimate body, you need to live a life that allows you to constantly be building and maintaining your work of art. This means changing your mentality from that of an out-of-shape dreamer into that of a disciplined, focused winner who is completely determined and self-confident. You have to want to be that person and want it bad.

You have to want to succeed badly enough to live into that person you want to be and keep achieving your goals your number-one priority. You need to accept that in order to get that amazing body you only see in 5 percent of the population, you will need to eat and train with a mind-set that 95 percent of the population does not hold. This involves discipline, consistency in training all muscle groups one to two times a week, with a minimum of three training sessions per week; proper diet and nutrition, consisting of honestly tracking calorie intake and macronutrient ratios (protein, fat, carbohydrates) based on your short-term goals of losing fat or building muscle; adequate hydration; and adequate sleep. This also involves limiting refined sugar, processed foods, alcohol, and in some cases carbohydrates in general.

You must be willing to commit to change and continue living this lifestyle for the foreseeable future. You are not only changing what you look like as a person; you are changing *who you are* as a person as well.

Your physical presence is your initial presentation to the rest of the world. What do you want them to take away from it? Your character, discipline, and self-worth are on display at first sight. Do they see a man or woman who holds him- or herself to a higher standard? A person who won't settle for a less-than-impressive physique? Or would they see the attributes of a person who is completely comfortable with mediocrity? Attractive women and men hold themselves to a higher standard that does not involve mediocrity. You want to be a woman or man who not only meets high personal expectations but raises the bar. You can get there. I can show you how. There are some major perks that go along with being in great shape.

GROW PHYSICALLY AND GROW MENTALLY

I HAVE PERSONALLY found that great muscle growth comes from perfect form, and the mind-muscle connection, which is basically the mental memorization of perfect form. The mental memorization of form is simply adjusting your body, based on wanting to achieve the exact angle at which the applied load is directly repelled away from or brought toward the body by the targeted muscle, as precisely as possible. For success in muscle growth, as it pertains to a well-detailed and proportionate physique, this must be a daily, ongoing process throughout your years of training. This is where weight training becomes psychological, and focus and control play a large role. It can take years of training for some individuals before they are able to properly focus their minds enough to feel the muscles they are trying to work.

Many people who I have spoken with, and the majority of people I see at the gym, are of the opinion that bodybuilding is a very simple hobby to partake in. I mean, really, how complicated is it? You walk up to a weight, lift it up a few times, and that's it, right? That's all there is to it. If you do that a bunch of times, you get strong, and if you do it a bunch more, you turn into the Terminator, right? It takes no brains or intellect; it takes no education or experience. That is the common belief. So many people I have seen in the gym throughout my years of working out, I would say around 90 percent, have no clue what it takes to reach the physique they desire. This is completely understandable, and I empathize with these people; I was once like them.

The weight room is very deceiving in its perceived simplicity. I too came from that state of mind where I believed that all there was to growing muscle was to lift a weight that used the muscle I wanted to grow, and if I kept doing that, I would reach my dream physique in no time. It only took me roughly fifteen years to figure out that this is not the case. Through an incredible amount of reading and continued persistence in training, I eventually came to realize that not only did I possess a minute fraction of what I needed to know for my goals, but I had wasted an incredible amount of time believing that I knew what I was doing and required no help or education from anyone else. I made this mistake, and a lot of people make it too. The major mistake was, I had no idea that I didn't know, and I thought I knew. A huge problem is that people think it is such an easy venture that they fail to educate themselves on the topic. They feel it is such a simple concept that they already know how to go about it and need not seek guidance or advice.

Even when people do decide to reach out and hire a trainer, the expectation of knowledge for a trainer to possess is incredibly low. Right now, the top certification company in Canada only requires a three-day in-class training session to become what they call a "personal training specialist." I have taken this course myself. The eleven other individuals in the class had no idea what they were doing when it came to weight training and were using this course as more of a situation of being trained by a personal trainer themselves, rather than already being competent and knowledgeable in the gym and using the course to show on paper that they knew their stuff. Not one person in that class of "personal training specialists" looked like he had ever even lifted anything, let alone a dumbbell or barbell. There was a portion of the course where we went to a fitness center that was attached to the classroom area and were supposed to be training a partner in common exercises that people use in the gym to work out. I was the only person in the class who could instruct the person I was working with on how to do the exercises properly. The other individuals had no idea what they were doing or what they were talking about. I am not saying this to brag or boast by any means. This is the reason why I want to put this information out and have it available to people. There are people who have a lot more knowledge on the subject than I will ever have. I just feel there is enough misinformation out there surrounding fitness and nutrition that I encourage anyone with real-world knowledge to put it out there and counteract this craziness that is going on these days.

Keep in mind that I have been interested in weight training and bodybuilding since I was very young. My parents bought me a beginner weight set one Christmas that consisted of three sets of dumbbells, two and a half, five, and ten pounds. I was only around ten years old at the time, and the interest snowballed form there. I seemed to be in my room alone a couple of times per week for disciplinary reasons, so experimenting with how my body worked under load was how I passed the time. When I started grade nine, my high school had just come out with a weight-training class, and I was very interested in any physical education for the sheer fact that it didn't bore me as much as math did. I ended up loving it and taking it every year, sometimes both semesters. I credit those classes and my teachers and trainers for most of my success, thanks to the knowledge they passed on.

My postsecondary education also involved fitness-training classes, so I continued learning throughout my college years. I then ended up being recruited by the military police, where I then *really* found out what limits I was able to push my mind and body to. This I have found to be an advantage, since through pushing my mind and body to extremes, I was able to expand what I believed was possible for my body to do. Breaking down barriers in your mind is of the utmost importance on your journey, whatever that journey may be.

There is no amount of teaching from a textbook or education that can replace the experience of twenty years in a gym, experimenting with your own body and pushing it to its limits. The fact that all these people are now certified personal trainers shows that there is an incredibly low expectation of what a personal trainer needs to accomplish in order to be paid. The expectation of the client doesn't make any sense to me. I believe it goes back to my previous statement that because success in weightlifting is so deceptive in appearing to be a very simple process, the expectation of knowledge and experience a trainer needs to possess must also be simple.

I assure you, it is not at all a simple process. It is, in fact, very complex. The amount of time it can take a person just to perform the exercise correctly is incredible. It is not as simple as walking into the gym, lying on a bench, and pressing the weight above your head ten times, then repeating that two more times. Reaching an incredible physique takes incredible knowledge of your own psychology and physiology. Lifting the weight is the simplest part of it. Your mind plays the major role. Your mind is what controls your body; your body does not control your mind. You have to dive deep into who you are as a person and how you are thinking every day in order to be successful.

When you see world-class bodybuilders, you see a physique that is incredible. When you see fitness models who are incredibly cut and aesthetic, it is an awe-inspiring thing to see the human body in such a way. What you aren't seeing, though, is what is going on behind the scenes. What you aren't seeing is the fact that in order to get those physiques that no one else has, they have had to train their minds just as much as their bodies to reach that higher state of thinking. They have to think the way no one else thinks, in order to reach heights no one else can reach. They have trained themselves to *think* in a way that others don't think. It takes incredible discipline, dedication, physical and mental fortitude, visualization, and belief in the unbelievable.

An area where many people get stuck wasting time when they begin is having the comparison mind-set. They look around the gym and start comparing what other people are doing to what they are doing. They start looking at how heavy the dumbbells are that they guy next to them is using or how much that person has loaded up on the bench press. I am not ashamed to say that I too once fell into this trap when I was starting out. It is human nature to protect our egos. I am telling you this because it can set you back *years* in your training. If you are always trying to appease your ego and are never lifting what you should be lifting for your abilities, you will never get a proper workout and never reach your potential. I have seen people much larger than me do routines with much less weight, and on the other end of the spectrum, I have seen much smaller people than me use a larger amount of weight for theirs. Everyone is different, and everyone's body has different capabilities and weaknesses. Your muscles may be working just as hard using a lighter weight as someone else using more weight. You will both be obtaining the same benefit and muscle growth from the workout; your muscle structure just differs slightly in the amount of weight needed to achieve it.

Everyone has a genetic potential that can eventually be reached. Some people's potential may be slightly higher or lower than yours, and there is nothing, aside from steroid use, that can take you past that point. There will come a day when you just can't increase the amount of weight you lift or the amount of muscle growth you get. If there were no limit, people would be bench pressing dump trucks in the parking lot.

(Though that does sound pretty cool.) That is not the only way the comparison mind-set will slow you down. If you walk into the gym and see a huge bodybuilder lifting a lot of weight, you may think you need to lift that amount of weight to look the way he does, but what about the other way around? If you walk in and see him with only thirty-five-pound plates on the bench press, what would you think then? Wouldn't common sense tell you he must have a strategy you know nothing about? Not all growth comes from lifting extreme weight. It can come from repetition as well.

Take tradesmen, for example. They do repetitive tasks all day, every day, and the result is usually a strength imbalance between appendages. The arm they use constantly to hold and use tools is usually significantly stronger than the non-dominant arm. The tools they use don't change in weight from day to day, but they still respond with growth. Weight does play a major role in pushing muscles to develop to their full potential, but it is not the only way growth can happen. Avoid comparing yourself to others in the gym. Other people are on their own paths with their own unique bodies. What they are doing has nothing to do with you and your goals, therefore it should not affect you.

There was a time when I believed that only people with a certain body type could ever have six-pack abs. I had convinced myself that it was impossible for me to ever achieve that. The reason I did this to myself was that it was easier to tell myself it was impossible than to admit that I hadn't really tried all that hard. I had to change my mind; I had to change my way of thinking and be completely honest with myself. I had to go deep into my mind and say to myself, "Admit it!" I didn't want to put in the effort. I was making excuses for my unwillingness to put in the work needed to get what I wanted. It was easier just to lie to myself and accept the lie than it was to properly educate myself and put what I needed to do into practice.

Finally, one day, I just made the decision to stop lying to myself, and I started to work on what I wanted. I reached a goal that I once believed was impossible for me to attain, all because I was able to look at my thought process as a conscious observer and find the fault that was holding me back. This is but one small example of how psychologically complex it can be to reach your physical goals. It takes incredible mental fortitude to push yourself through years of training; to fail at what you are doing; to feel that you have wasted time working toward something when you don't see the results you were expecting; giving up and failing, and then deciding to start again and repeating that process multiple times, as I have done.

There have been years when I have given up trying to reach my desired physique. I have given up on dieting at times, for the mere fact that I simply was just not yet strong enough mentally to continue putting myself through the struggle. I have had to convince myself on multiple occasions to get back to it; get back on it and keep going; get myself back in the gym, start from zero again, get back to where I was, and make it past the point where I gave up last time. I have failed multiple times, over and over, but every time I failed, I learned something new. There is so much in training that derives from within your mind that simply cannot be taught in a classroom. It simply can only be experienced. That is why it is so crucial to your success to find someone who has been through this process. Not someone who has taken a postsecondary diploma or degree program or a three-day personal-training course. You need to find someone who not only can guide you in the gym but can guide you to finding yourself mentally. Someone who can help you unlock those thoughts and limiting beliefs you have formed in your mind, recognize them, and push you past them in order to reach your ultimate potential.

The spectrum of experience and competence in personal trainers is so incredibly vast that I do not envy anyone who is currently partaking in the search for the one who will make the difference between success and failure. If you are not careful with whom you trust, you could end up making a very poor financial investment and, even worse, wasting months of possible gain. For beginners who are just starting on their path, personal training is your best bet at success. But finding the right one is crucial. If you want to take twenty-five-plus years to figure out how to develop your body on your own, I'm sure it is possible to learn through trial and error yourself, but for anyone who is serious about reaching an unmatched physical presence and favors personal time and money, seeking out those who have already acquired the knowledge and experience you need to get whatever you want is common sense.

A trainer who has proven success personally is unmatched by any textbook-only, two-year-diploma type of trainer. Real, experienced trainers are the ultimate resource for cutting the time it will take you to reach your desired physique down to a minimum. Trainers are by no means needed for everyone's entire journey, but for getting started, proper instruction and training examples are definitely crucial to timely success. Your trainer should resemble someone close to who you want to be, someone who has reached similar goals; someone who is training because they truly love what training has done for their life and wants to help others achieve the same success. Not someone who took a two-year college diploma or a three-day certification course because the early-childhood education course was full. Someone who has achieved the goals you are setting for yourself and understands what needs to be done to reach them.

When it comes to fitness and bodybuilding, there is no formal education that can replace experience working your guts out in the gym and experimenting with calorie intake and macronutrients, which I have been doing now for twenty years. When I train a person, it involves life coaching for mental strength as well as physical fitness. Not only do you need to elevate your physical capacity for workouts, but you need to strengthen your mind and elevate it to a new way of looking at your life, to really get on that level you want to be on. I help people who have guts, determination, and drive; who want to do what most people think is impossible. I want to show people how to develop into the person they have always felt they were. Be a person others look at with lust and awe; a person who makes others think twice about the type of man or woman they chose as a partner; a person other people look at with envy. When you look good and feel good, the confidence and discipline you develop will attract success from all avenues.

WHAT, AND HOW I EAT TO LOOK GREAT

Nutrition is the hardest part. Without eating properly for your goals, your efforts are useless. Period. I have seen individuals in the gym look the same for years, despite being consistent in their workouts and working their asses off—because they simply don't know how, or they are unwilling to eat for their desired physique. The old saying, "You can't outtrain a bad diet," says it best. No matter how hard you work or how consistent you are, if you are not eating right, you will see very little change in your body. The examples of eating I give in this section are based on my own body type, mesomorph. I have no issues gaining muscle (and fat) on a fairly low-calorie count, around twenty-five hundred calories, for example, since my metabolism is relatively middle ground. However, this means that when it comes to fat loss, my calorie intake will also be fairly low, which can make dieting quite challenging.

If you are an ectomorph, you will have the opposite struggles. Being naturally lean, your metabolism is quite high, so you will be able to lose fat while keeping your calorie count fairly high. Eating enough calories to gain muscle during a bulking phase will likely be your challenge. When reading information on dieting and caloric intake, it is important to know the background and body type of the individual you are getting the information from. If they started out naturally thin with a low body fat percentage, their information on losing body fat may be a bit less reliable than someone who came from being overweight. Someone's suggestions on muscle gain may, on the other hand, be less reliable if that person started off with natural size and strength. Make sure your sources are sound, and don't put all your eggs in one basket.

Beginners can make the mistake of thinking this is not the case, because if you have never weight trained before, you will see *some* change in your physique just from starting, but soon after, your progress will grind to a quick halt and become stagnant. This is from your body just adjusting to the new loads you are placing on it. If you want to take your body to the next level, you will need to begin eating like you want to get there. But, like anything, the more you do it, the better you will get at it. Some will have issues with eating too much, and some will have issues with not eating enough. Some will have issues giving up daily refined sugar.

Dieting is very closely related to other human tendencies that involve benefiting from self-restraint, like recovering drug addicts or compulsive gamblers. They all involve instant gratification and the Hedonic Response, which is a psychological tendency of the brain to desire pleasure and avoid discomfort or pain. Our brains have evolved to keep us comfortable and avoid anything else. So, if instant gratification is available to us, be it painkilling drugs, the adrenaline rush of placing a bet, or the sexual arousal provided by pornography available at our fingertips, in order to grow or develop past this constant indulgence of instant gratification, we must take control of our minds and force the self-control on ourselves if we want to progress in our goals. Therefore, hedonic hunger would be eating for pleasure, instead of eating to sustain the energy and nutrient needs of the body. This phenomenon can be brought on by simply thinking about food that you find pleasurable. Hunger itself can be brought on purely by thinking about food. This hedonic response is very closely related to sex and can be extremely intense. Hedonic hunger can be equated to sexual arousal. The arousal is the sheer anticipation or consideration of sexual experience. Think of how much self-control you would need not to partake with your ideal sexual partner and pull away at the height of arousal. For most people who have never attempted this experiment, it may seem to be the hardest thing they used their minds to attempt, no pun intended.

It is very important to realize how the mind works in order to reach your goals and that it is in fact your *mind,* not only *your* mind, but everyone's mind that operates like this. If you do practice these restraints, you will eventually seize control over your mind and your actions. Self-control is thought control. If you can control your mind, you can control your actions. This is where I speak as a male, frankly because I am one. If you practice self-restraint in regards to masturbation for instance, you will instantly reap the rewards. Our bodies are designed to seek every avenue that will result in procreation. When you abstain from sex, your body will heighten everything in your ability, in order to get you closer to attract and procreate with a female. You are more driven to succeed. You are naturally more confident in your daily activities. You carry yourself with more assurance and move thorough your day with more purpose and aggression. I am not speaking about becoming a monk or any sense of extremism here. It is only my opinion that if you have a task in front of you that requires aggressive focus and want a slight edge when it comes to confidence and determination, try periods of abstinence and observe how you operate closely.

Your body naturally creates more testosterone, which is the hormone that pushes you into this heightened state of seek and destroy. Studies have proven that the longer men go without sexual release, the higher their testosterone levels go, until they reach their peak. If you are, as Jerry Seinfeld says, "master of your domain," you are actually the master of your mind, and moving quicker toward your goals and your successes. Simply by abstaining from self-gratification for prolonged periods of time, you instantly create a level of advantage for yourself.

You are not the only one who must struggle in order to overcome the natural tendencies of the human condition. Every successful person in the world has had to overcome first before achieving his or her level of success. In regards to dieting, though, genetics and eating disorders can play a role in some cases, to what level this occurs, but for the otherwise-healthy individual, it is able to be recognized and conquered like anything else. These are examples that conclude that a lot of people seem to think that they have utilized a good amount off control in their life, that they have a good grip on self-control and are directing their life as they want. In reality, most people are *not* in control, and when tested under serious circumstances, they will fail unless they have worked and practiced this skill.

Think of it this way. Many people know how to cook, but we rely on the ease of having a stove, electricity, a frying pan, or a grill. What would happen if we were in a situation where we were starving to death and none of these things existed? If you were Survivor-Man, (shout out, by the way, love you, Les Stroud, you da man!) say you had practiced being in this situation over and over and been successful. You would likely come out all right. If you had never practiced being in this situation and had never successfully forced yourself to adapt, the chances of your survival would be minimal at best. The same thing goes for dieting. The more you put yourself in that situation, the more you are going to learn how to adapt, using different strategies to help you complete each goal. Find fuel, light the fire, make a spit, and so on.

Yes, the first scenario you ever try will be the worst. Your wood may be green, you may not be able to find a spark, and your meat may be covered in grass and sand, but unlike survival, you will have the chance for a mulligan. You are allowed as many as you need in order to succeed one day. The only way you can fail is if you stop trying. When you do succeed and you have met your goal, even if you regress, you will have a fundamental advantage over others who have not yet succeeded. You have now seen that your faith in what you were practicing worked! All that discipline and all that effort worked. You didn't do it for nothing. So now you know that if you continue to put in that game plan, your results are guaranteed. There is no more believing in the unseen. Being able to know with certainty that the suffering you are enduring will produce the results you want is much different than having to go on trust alone. Once you reach that first goal, your certainty in your ability to obtain that level can never diminish, and it will be a huge step in changing you into the person you want to become.

Proper dieting consists of setting a specific goal of either losing fat (cutting) or building muscle (bulking). I personally recommend cutting first, because with a layer of fat on your body, you will not see the muscle gains you are making underneath. If you are already very low in body fat, this is not a concern for you, and you will go right into bulking. Start off by counting your calories. *Every calorie*, from the cream in your coffee to the mustard on your sandwich. Using a food scale is the only way to track your calories accurately. This will allow you to learn exactly the amount you are eating and adjust it to your goals. The app My Fitness Pal is what I personally use and recommend. It is a free, simple-to-use phone application that makes calorie counting much easier.

Once you have figured out how to count your calories, you will need to figure out your basal metabolic rate or BMR. This is the "maintenance" amount of calories your body needs to sustain itself, neither burning fat nor building muscle, for one day with no added exercise. Bulking will involve eating five hundred to seven hundred calories over your BMR or maintenance amount, and cutting will involve eating five hundred to seven hundred calories under your maintenance amount. Once you have your target calorie amount, you will then start to track your macronutrients or proteins, fats, and carbohydrates. Specific ratios are needed to obtain your ultimate goal physique. For example, while in a cutting phase, I aim to eat my body weight in grams of protein daily and fill in the rest with fats and carbohydrates. My macro ratios look like this: 50 percent protein, 35 percent carbs, 15 percent fat. This is a good starting point, and it is not written in stone either. I have gone through cutting phases that provided excellent results eating as low as three-fourths of my body weight in protein as well. While bulking, my calories increase, but my macronutrient ratios stay pretty similar.

While cutting, you need to be very precise, as every calorie counts. While bulking, you are able to relax just a bit and not be as strict on every number. However, your results will still depend on your discipline. For example, if you still don't consume enough carbohydrates while bulking and you only eat fat and protein, you may not get the intended results based on your body type. You may still grow, but you could be growing faster if you hit your nutritional needs. Most people will need to adjust their calories and macro ratios for how their body uses each one, based on their personal metabolism. There are minor differences for everyone, but start with gaining the knowledge of what you are aiming for first. Schedule yourself at least one cheat day every seven days. This will help you keep your sanity, and you will likely feel so gross afterward that you will be very happy to be back to eating properly the following week. Having a cheat day will also be restoring your body's metabolism to full swing by telling your body it's OK to lose more fat, because food is readily available.

Too much of anything can be bad, and that includes calorie restriction. If you are on a very low calorie count, having a cheat day when you eat a lot of calories and carbohydrates can also allow your body to replenish any energy or nutrient stores it is lacking. My advice would be to try not to go too crazy, and try to ensure you still get your protein intake for the day. The chaos that a cheat day initiates in your body is a good thing to keep it guessing and adjusting. A common practice of mine is if I find that I have indulged in a lot of carbohydrates on a cheat day, which is often the case, the next day I will abstain from carbs completely on my first day back to my normal eating habits. For example, if I have a cheat day on a Sunday, I will then ensure I eat between twenty and fifty grams of carbohydrates on the following Monday. I will not normalize my carbohydrate intake until Tuesday at 3:00 p.m. This ensures that any excess glycogen that I built up in my system is burned off completely and not stored as fat.

There are so many people pushing so many gimmicky diets and eating styles these days for marketing purposes, it is getting completely out of control. Most of these marketers have an agenda to sell you on thoughts and ideas you do not need. I have experimented with various diets and eating styles, simply for my own interest and to try new suggestions along my path. I have done paleo, keto, Atkins, low-carb, intermittent fasting, just to name a few, and have found that no one diet will offer you the results you are looking for. But I also have learned that educating yourself and attempting different eating habits will result in a lot of knowledge and experience on how the human body operates as a result of what you put in it.

I have gained an enormous amount of nutritional information, just by trying these different diets, but I have found that they are all just a lot of hype. Your eating can be simplified into just knowing your daily calorie requirement to maintain your weight. If you want to lose fat, stay below that amount. If you want to gain muscle, stay slightly above that amount. Ensure you are at least reaching your daily requirement of protein. Eat whole foods like chicken, beef, eggs, cheese, fruits, and vegetables, and stay away from processed starches and simple processed sugars. Eat your carbohydrates around your workouts whenever possible, and drink plenty of water. It's really that simple.

I have also found that when you are eating in a calorie deficit, one very beneficial eating style to practice is intermittent fasting. This one is real, folks. The practice of fasting has been proven to provide significant health benefits for the human body. The benefits I receive are a faster rate of fat loss, greater concentration ability, and clarity of thought, especially in the morning; lower water retention, greater overall energy, lower blood pressure and pulse, to name the ones right off the top of my head. So really, I find this practice not only very beneficial to staying within my calorie count, since I eat all my calories in an eight-hour window of time, which allows me to be satiated for a period of time every day, but very beneficial to my clarity of thought and my energy levels early in the day. Intermittent fasting has been shown to lower blood-glucose and insulin levels, which would facilitate greater fat loss. Production of human growth hormone is increased, which facilitates muscle growth and fat burning. It has been found to promote greater efficiency in cellular repair and toxin removal. Studies in rats show that fasting may increase growth of new nerve cells, which would provide benefits for increased brain function. It also increases levels of a brain hormone called brain-derived neurotrophic factor (BDNF). A deficiency in BDNF has been associated with depression as well as other impaired brain functionalities.

A study published by Louisiana State University Medical Center in 2007 resulted in the finding that alternate-day fasting provides relief for asthma symptoms, inflammation, and oxidative stress in asthma patients who were overweight.

Experimental studies in animals have shown that intermittent fasting reduces the risk of diabetes and lowers blood pressure, triglyceride levels, and cholesterol. The US National Institute on Aging published a study that found that in rats, alternate-day fasting defended the brain cells from toxins, protected against damage from stroke, and showed a slowed cognitive decline in mice specifically bred to develop Alzheimer's disease.

In 2016, Yoshinori Ohsumi was awarded the Nobel Prize in Physiology/Medicine for his findings of mechanisms for autophagy. This is a process the body uses to remove and recycle damaged protein in brain cells. Intermittent fasting has been shown in animal studies to speed up the autophagy process. This process is activated by cell starvation. Disruption in the autophagy process has been linked to diseases such as Parkinson's and type-2 diabetes, as well as other disorders that usually appear in later in life with the elderly. The mutations in autophagy genes are also believed to contribute to the formation of cancer and other genetic diseases such as Alzheimer's disease.

I currently fast from 11:00 p.m. to 3:00 p.m. the next day, sixteen hours in total. I have also found that my fat-loss results are heightened if I can extend the fast to eighteen or twenty hours or more. Eating your daily calorie content in an eight-hour period allows you the ability to feel full and satiated every day for that eight-hour period. The first few attempts at this eating style will take some getting used to, but your body will adapt, and it will eventually become your norm. Even after learning about all these benefits and feeling them work for me in my own body, the real reason I practice this eating method is that it makes cutting calories *so much easier!* I start the first half of the day feeling great, full of energy and clarity of thought, with a little bit of hunger starting in the afternoon. Then I get to eat eighteen hundred calories in an eight-hour period, so I am full for half the day as well. The health benefits are awesome, but that is the real reason I use it.

A trick I use if I feel a bit hungry is taking a swig of apple-cider vinegar with a glass of water. I find it takes my appetite away for a couple of hours. I'm not sure if this is just me, but it works. It actually also has its own health benefits, which is what started me taking it. Then I found that was an added benefit to it. Sipping on black coffee or sparkling water can also be great. Sugar-free carbonated drinks keep you feeling full and can really help you make it through those last couple hours if you are a beginner.

Remember, you have to do what others are unwilling to do in order to get what others don't have. Think differently than the masses to reach places the masses can't get to.

These days you can't even browse the Internet without coming across at least some type of supplement. It is a multibillion-dollar industry that relies on mass confusion, misinformation, and overhyped products and ingredients. I would hazard a guess that if you are going the natural route, you don't need 98 percent of what is being marketed out there, if any at all. All the nutrients you need are available in your food. The only supplement I currently use is creatine monohydrate. It is the most-researched supplement out there other than protein. I find I have no problem getting all the protein I need from my food sources, and I feel much better when I don't use the processed jar crud unless absolutely necessary. If I was in a serious time crunch or unable to find a natural whole-food protein source, I would cave, but only under duress. Other supplements that may be of use to a few individuals would be weight gainers or mass gainers if you are naturally lean as hell and finding you have an insanely high metabolism and need to eat a ridiculous amount of food to put on any size at all. If you are not an ectomorph, you don't need them.

Chances are, if you are a mesomorph or endomorph and you start consuming weight gainers, you will just end up gaining significantly more fat than muscle. Just consume as much whole natural food as possible, and all the nutrients you need will be readily available. Relying on supplements to get you through your workout and diet is simply a crutch. You don't need a crutch. All you need is a strong drive and desire to reach your goals. I used to use preworkouts for a while but found they eventually caused me more distress than assistance. The amounts of caffeine and other drugs in some preworkouts would leave me feeling agitated and irritable after they wore off. I found I would be restless and unable to get a good night's sleep while using them, so I stopped. The strain they caused on my mind outweighed the very temporary benefits I would get. After a while, I became addicted to their use, and my mind started to believe I wouldn't be able to get through my workouts without them. There is a time and a place where a preworkout could be beneficial to some people who work long hours or are up very early in the morning with little sleep. All I am saying is that, for me, I don't find they really benefit me enough to use them, and I would avoid relying on anything other than your mind to get that aggression in your gym time.

I personally don't need to rely on anything but myself to get me through my workouts and keep me focused on my goals. However, my morning cup of Tim Hortons doesn't hurt either. Right now, as I type this, all I use is creatine monohydrate. There is proven scientific evidence that shows creatine improves performance in high-intensity, short-burst aerobic exercise. However, do your own research. It is still a dietary supplement and should be used only by healthy adults over eighteen. If you have any health concerns, do not use *any* supplement without talking to your doctor

———

In my twenty years of use, I personally have never experienced any side-effects and have found that taking five grams of creatine daily after my workouts provides a significant increase in strength and is very noticeable during heavy sets. As creatine increases water retention in muscle tissue, it is important that you consume ample amounts of water to ensure proper hydration is met for your entire system.

Really, no one absolutely *needs* supplements, so you can save your cash and still get shredded as hell. Spend that hundred bucks you were going to spend on protein and preworkouts and treat yourself to whole unprocessed shrimp, chicken, steak, and a good cup of coffee instead, and you will feel much better than relying on processed pharmaceutical cocktails. Although I say you don't absolutely need to spend money on supplements, I do have my own personal selection of products I have found to be useful in helping me to reach my goals, but this book is not for pushing products. This book is for you to get the facts about what you can do on your own, with your own mind, eating real food. There is no magic pill out there, so be careful before giving up your hard-earned money for minuscule benefits.

The supplement industry has been able to grow to such epic proportions largely due to flaws in human psychology. People want to believe there is an excuse for failing to achieve their goals. It's not their fault. There must be another reason why they haven't achieved what they set out to do. It can't just be that they aren't doing what they really need to be doing or that they just aren't working hard enough at eating properly. No, it must be a lack of protein or amino acids, or not enough caffeine or not enough vitamins or low testosterone. They also want a short cut to success. It's just human nature. But how much money are people going to spend to realize that no matter how flashy the label, no matter which model is on the front or who the spokesperson is, nothing, I repeat *nothing* you can buy in a store will replace the time, effort, and intensity you will have to give in the gym to take the micro-advantages they are claiming to offer you?

There are no short cuts to success. Success only comes from taking every minute in the day and trying to make them all count for you. If you want the muscles, nothing is going to lift that weight for you. *You* actually have to lift that weight and go through the pain of tearing down your muscles and then eating the right nutrients to rebuild them in the most efficient way possible. No supplement is going to do that for you. There are no such things as overnight successes. Successes take a long time to achieve. You make your plan, you belly up to it, and you go all in; that's how you succeed. Like I said before, be dangerous—in business, in the gym, in life. The most dangerous people in life are the ones who are willing to fight like they have nothing left to lose.

Here's a good analogy to consider for personal training. If you are looking to build a house and you don't want to build a house that looks exactly the same as everyone else's house, what do you do? You have to hire a custom architect. You need to seek someone out who has the specialized knowledge on how to go about building something just for you the way you want it. Chances are, if you are looking for a house no one else has, you need to seek out someone who can show you options no one else is using. Usually, people abstain from this choice, as customization usually comes at a premium cost; you are paying for the fact that there is a limited supply of designers who can produce the product you desire. It is simply supply and demand. There are only a few people who can design and build a custom home, but there are many people who can produce houses that are identical to all the others. The custom-home designer may require more time and specialty techniques, but the result is a product that is completely unique.

HOW TO LOSE EIGHT POUNDS OF WATER IN ONE AND A HALF DAYS

When you have a cheat day, what do most people crave? Carbohydrates, mostly. I personally can gain up to ten pounds from one day of unrestricted carbohydrate intake, most of which is water retention, since you store roughly three grams of water for every gram of carbohydrate you consume. Here is my method for losing that water weight in a day and a half. First, I usually end my cheat day around 7:00 p.m. The next day is crucial. I make sure I do an extended cardio session that includes high-intensity interval training and get a good sweat going on. The more I sweat, the better. My weight-training session I also keep quite intense, as I have the energy from the excess carbohydrates to sustain it. Again, the more sweat, the better. Catching on yet? I then take either a hot shower for ten minutes or sit in the steam room for ten to fifteen minutes. The longer, the better, but I don't always have all day to sit in the steam room or sauna. The more sweat you can get dripping off you the better.

I constantly drink water and cold tea (green or orange pekoe) with lemon. I will consume around eight liters of water throughout the day, frequently urinating all day long. The following day, I practice intermittent fasting and fast until 7:00 p.m. That's right, that is a twenty-four-hour fast. If you are versed in intermittent fasting, your body gets used to it, and after a cheat day, it is very easy to go twenty-four hours with no food. I then restrict myself to just eight hundred calories for that day and cut out all carbohydrates other than what exist naturally in my vegetables. I eat a small meal of vegetables only around 7:00 p.m., and I eat another portion of fats, protein, and vegetables around one hour before I go to bed, but not past 11:00 p.m., since I fast for sixteen hours, 11:00 p.m. to 3:00 p.m. the next day.

The next day, I again do not consume any food until 3:00 p.m. At this time, I return to my regular calorie and macro (carb) intake for my goals and continue on training. This usually will bring me down at least eight pounds, if not more, and bring me very close to where I was before I started my cheating. This is something that I had to experiment with on my own body. This is simply how I achieve it and what has worked for me. There are no guarantees that this process will work for you or is healthy for you personally. I am not a nutritionist or a doctor. I speak only from my own personal experiences. This is simply an example of the experimentation that needs to be done with your own body in order to understand how it works. If you are planning on restricting your calories to a very low level, I would suggest talking with your doctor first and having a physical exam done with bloodwork, to make sure everything is in order and you aren't going to put your body in jeopardy doing something drastic.

One of the first places anyone looks for information is online. The Internet is an incredible source of information for anyone seeking knowledge on a specific topic. However, with fitness and nutrition, there is just as much misleading, incorrect information out there as there is correct and factual information that is backed up by scientific study and evidence. It can be very hard as a beginner or someone who has not yet met desired goals to decipher and sort through the millions of articles, blogs, and forums found on the topic online. Your best source is to go old school. Yep, you're going to have to socialize. Your best source of information is going to be real life. Get off the Internet and go and find someone who is reaching your goals or who has met them in the past. Go to the gym, go to a natural-physique competition, go to a fitness expo, or find a trainer who coaches physique athletes. Yes, there are some individuals on YouTube that know their stuff, and yes, they can be helpful, but finding someone in real life who has no agenda, no products to push, and no supplement company would pretty much guarantee that if they are willing to give you some tips, they are being honest and up front with you. Ask them where they started, what they looked like; were they fat, were they skinny, did they have a hard time building muscle or losing fat? Were they very weak, or have they always been strong? Have they always had a genetic advantage in a specific part of the body like huge triceps or a wide back? The best way to know what you have to do is to find someone who has come from the same place you are now and been able to get to where they are now.

If you can find someone who is a close match for you genetically, that information is priceless, and you should be willing to pay them for it 100 percent. Most of the people out there who are writing blogs or commenting in forums really have no idea what they are talking about, and it shows. A lot of people I see commenting on forums are just spouting information that they read somewhere else online that is inaccurate or only accurate for certain individuals with specific genetics. Anyone who has reached the desired physique or very close to it has an easier time picking out this nonsense, since they know what has worked and what does work as well as what does not. They have put in the time and the trial and error and patience with their diet, testing different info and experimenting with different macronutrient percentages and meal timing. If you have not yet done that, it would be almost impossible for you to get all the information you require for yourself from one source. I personally have experimented with various diets, meal timings, eating styles, training methods, and cardio routines.

The conclusion I would love to share with you is that there is no one diet, method, or ratio that works best for everyone. You just need to try them all. That's right. Go and try them. Go paleo for six months, go keto for six months, go Atkins, go vegan. The more you try, the more you learn. Read about all of them. Then keep track either mentally or in a journal of what your body does during that time. How did you feel pre- and post-workout? How did you feel in the morning, and how did you feel at nighttime before bed? Did you have more energy at times and less at others? Did you lose fat quickly, or did you get stronger in certain areas? What was your overall state of mind? Were you happy or irritable? Did you have clarity of thought, or were you groggy and wanting to nap all the time? Keep track of all of this. I have developed my current eating habits based on everything I kept note of while doing different diets and utilizing different calorie amounts and macronutrient ratios.

Take all of the knowledge you have gained from going through this process, and pick out the parts that benefitted you the most. The reason I eat what I eat and when is because that is what I found worked the best for me. I don't know if that's what works for everyone, so I can't sit here and say you have to do this this and this at this time or else. There are people who can eat as many carbs as they want and still not gain an ounce of fat when they bulk. I, however, gain fat really quickly the higher my carb consumption is, but at the same time, I feel like utter garbage for months on end if I don't, so I have based my carb count on that information. There is absolutely no other way for me personally to gain that information about myself without putting my body through time when I feel like utter crap on less than 150 grams of carbs per day, even when I was doing the ketogenic diet, which puts your body into a state called ketosis where it is running on ketones instead of blood glucose formed by carbohydrates. This allows the body to burn stored body fat as its main source of energy. But even through this, I found I still was lacking energy, even after being on this diet for months with very low carbs. I am talking less than twenty grams per day. I just felt like garbage, not only energy-wise but mentally I just wasn't well. I just didn't *feel* good. Yes, I did lose fat, and yes, it definitely does work. But for me and for a large part of the medical society, the jury is still out on whether it is the best option for otherwise-healthy individuals.

So, from this, depending on how I feel while I'm cutting, I now may go up to two hundred grams of carbohydrates in a day, which for me is high, since my total calorie intake while cutting is eighteen hundred calories on days I work out. If I'm not in the gym that day, I keep it at fifteen hundred. Sometimes toward the end of my training sessions for the week, I get that feeling I know very well, when I can feel my body is short on carbs. I have worked off the carbohydrates I need faster than usual for whatever reason that week, and I know I need to adjust my carb count a bit higher for the last couple of days of the week. I keep my calories the same, but I steal a few from fat to add in the carbohydrates. That is knowledge only personal experimentation can produce, and it's up to you to keep a record of it. If you can't do it in your head, buy a simple notebook or keep track on your phone in an app.

If you happen to find yourself browsing forums and information online, remember there are definitely some fundamental understandings that people with proven results agree on.

1. Best results, for fat loss or muscle gain, come from a high-protein diet.
2. In order to gain muscle mass, you need a caloric surplus.
3. In order to lose fat, you need a caloric deficit.

If you come across any information that goes against these three fundamentals, be extremely skeptical of it. As for carbohydrate intake, there are still very substantiated arguments on both sides of the fence. But what I can tell you is I am no doctor, nutritionist, or scientist, but I feel my best mentally and physically when I have a portion of my diet include carbohydrates. However, the type of carbs definitely makes all the difference in the world. You just can't expect that a donut with icing on it, a chemically concocted dreamboat of a treat and one of my favorites, would have the same nutritional value to your system as a natural piece of fresh fruit, for example. That is just pure sense. Not only is it more beneficial to your overall growth and development, but the fiber content in fruit as well as whole grains keeps you feeling full longer than simple sugars do, so you are less likely to relapse into a downward spiral of sugar-induced insanity. Fiber also helps your body regulate insulin levels, which determine the rate at which to process blood sugar and store fat.

The fiber in fruit slows the digestion of sugar. You may find people who talk about IIFYM (if it fits your macros) habits of eating whatever they want, as long as their macro nutrients stay the same. For instance, they believe that if you are limited to three hundred grams of carbs in a day, it doesn't make a difference whether those carbs come from a chocolate bar, pizza dough, or a banana. Yes, your body may utilize the carbs, especially in those people who have high metabolisms and are naturally lean; you won't instantly gain fat from them, but do you *really* think your body uses processed, refined sugar the same way it would use a nutrient-dense, natural piece of organic fruit? There is definitely a lot of ignoring common sense and scientific evidence to convince yourself that thinking would be accurate.

Do not make excuses. If you want to reach your goals faster, eat your sweets responsibly on a planned cheat day, and don't go too crazy! Other than that, opt for low-glycemic carbohydrates. Whole grains, fruits, nuts, dairy, and vegetables are what you want if you want to optimize your heath and your road to victory. There is absolutely nothing wrong with sugar from fresh, natural fruit; it is full of nutrients and fiber and perfect for pre- and postworkout carb source, since it contains simple sugars like glucose, fructose, and sucrose that are absorbed very quickly by the body after exercise. If you consume too much sugar or quick-digesting simple carbs while inactive and in a calorie surplus, that sugar will be stored in the liver. Once the liver is full, that sugar will be turned into fatty acids that will travel in your blood, right to your love handles. So eat your simple carbs around your workouts, and keep the amount in check. I personally eat 30 to 50 grams of simple carbohydrates from fresh fruit postworkout. Most days I eat around 150 to 170 grams of carbohydrates while cutting, so 30 to 50 grams would be about a third of my total carbs for the day. Remember, this is just what I do. Use it as a suggested starting point; don't start a religion on it.

PART - BEGINNER BASICS FOR MUSCLE DEVELOPMENT

SIMPLY PUT, AGAIN, I know this is frustrating to hear, but truly, there is no short cut to success. You have to be willing to put in the work. If you are at the point where you are about ready to give up, don't let this stop you. You can't quit now! Sometimes you may not be able to see your progress visually. You just have to keep the faith and stay the course. When you are gaining muscle or losing weight, sometimes your body may appear as if it is not changing. You may not be able to see any progress for weeks at a time, then all of a sudden, bam! One morning, you wake up and you see a couple of creases in your abdominals, or your shoulders that weren't there yesterday. You just have to trust that what you desire is coming to you through your continued efforts and patience. You have just gained all this knowledge and are doing the right thing by continuing to seek it out!

But unfortunately, your work doesn't end when you leave the gym for the day. In fact, I find the hardest work is done outside the gym in the day-to-day moments when you are learning through not getting the results you desire and starting again. *That* is the real hard part, which played a major part in my wanting to share this information with others—*not* giving up. Not stopping at one month of feeling like you have made no progress. Not stopping after falling off the wagon. Not stopping at feeling like shit. And not stopping while trying to reach your goals and balance all the other aspects that have nothing to do with this in this crazy thing we call life. If you want to get to where you know you want to be, accept the failure as knowledge gained, stop being a bitch, and get the fuck back to work.

Here are my five steps for beginning muscle growth, regardless of what muscle is being trained:

STEP #1-LEARN CORRECT FORM

Great muscle growth comes from perfect form and the mind-muscle connection, which is basically the mental memorization of perfect form. The mental memorization of form is simply adjusting your body based on wanting to achieve the exact angle at which the applied load is directly repelled away from or brought toward the body by the targeted muscle, as precisely as possible.

STEP #2-FOCUS ON CONNECTING YOUR MIND TO YOUR MUSCLE

Focus your mind on what muscles you are feeling under the load of the weight; bring the weight all the way down or back, and feel those muscles stretch. Allow the pause all the time at the bottom of the rep, and feel the stretch. Do this with your eyes closed for a greater sensory experience. Is it the muscle you are targeting stretching, or is it another muscle group? If it is not your targeted muscle, adjust the angle slightly and do another repetition. Repeat this process until you have been able to stretch the targeted muscle repeatedly and can find it every time. If you are doing bench press, that would be a "push" movement, and the stretch would come from lowering the weight toward your chest. If you are doing a "pull" movement like seated cable rows, the stretch would come from allowing the weight to be drawn away from you.

STEP #3-UP THE WEIGHT

Up the weight slowly, as I said, no ego lifting! No one who is focused on their goals cares what you are doing anyway. Half the reps will get you half the gains. You should be able to use perfect form, stretching with a slight pause at the bottom for eight to twelve repetitions. If you fail at twelve, add weight until you fail at eight. If you fail at eight, keep doing sets at this weight until you are able to reach twelve three times. If you can only do four or six, lower the weight until you can at least do a set of eight with proper form.

STEP #4-UP THE INTENSITY (LESS REST BETWEEN SETS) INTERMEDIATE/ADVANCED

If you have been doing sets of eight repetitions with the same weight for six months, I think it's time to check your intensity. Try different (harder) exercises, up the weight, or add a variable like chains or weight belts to your exercises that need it.

STEP #5-UP THE VOLUME-INTERMEDIATE/ADVANCED

Very simply, add more sets. I like to do routines where I will do six sets at times. Sets one to two will be of lower repetitions at higher weight, and sets three to six will be of higher repetitions at lower weight. I also like to add in extra exercises, four chest exercises or five back exercises, to ensure I really exhaust the muscles. I do this based on how I feel the intensity of my workout has been. For example, if I am on my third exercise, and I have really been on the nose with intensity, I will be satisfied not going on to the fourth exercise. I will sometimes also use this trick if I feel I am falling behind in the development of a certain muscle I want to bring up to par. The most significant changes I saw in my physique came from increasing the volume during my routines. That means more sets, more reps. I start an exercise off with heavy weight and end with light weight. For my last three sets, I focus on getting as much of a "pump" as possible. If, for example, you aren't walking away from your chest routine feeling like you've increased two cup sizes, get back on the bench and grow those pecs.

Now let's move on to the meat and potatoes, the muscle groups. Unfortunately, reading is not going to do much in the way of helping you to actually perform these exercises. You need to get into the gym and experience it yourself. Instructional videos are the next-best thing to being in the gym yourself.

Chest—Either every guy's favorite, or if they have good leg genetics and not-so-good chest genetics, their secret favorite. One recommendation is to hit chest on a day other than Monday. Mondays are also known in the fitness world as International Chest Day. Since it's most male's favorite exercise, it's the first one they often hit when getting back into the gym on a Monday. If you walk into a gym between four and five on a weekday afternoon, chances are you're going to be waiting in line to get on a bench press.

Training chest properly and completely involves the training and development of the entire pectoralis muscle. The pec muscle needs to be hit from various angles to ensure full development. This is the reason for the change in angle you see on the benches. The more upright you are sitting, the more of the upper portion of the chest is targeted, as well as the front of the shoulder (anterior deltoid) as a secondary. The most common exercises utilize incline, flat, and decline benches, coupled with dumbbell and barbell movements. There are many various exercises that can complement a chest routine, such as body weight or weighted dips, cable work, and other more advanced training methods.

However, it is imperative that beginners learn the basic fundamental exercises that have been proven to give the most overall growth and development before experimenting with secondary, isolating exercises in order to properly maximize their potential for future success in their training.

These primary movements can be done with either dumbbells or barbells, but my recommendation is to try both initially, see which one you most like the feeling of, commit to fully learning and understanding the movement, and utilize it for at least ninety days of training before making the switch and trying the other in the same fashion. This will allow you to focus on the mind-muscle connection and allow for the first stages of mentally memorizing the proper form needed to get the best contraction that, in turn, allows for the best pump and ultimately the most growth.

As previously stated in the introduction, the mental memorization of form is simply adjusting your body based on wanting to achieve the exact angle at which the applied load is directly repelled away from or brought toward the body by the targeted muscle as precisely as possible. For success in muscle growth as it pertains to a well-detailed and proportionate physique, this must be an ongoing learning process throughout your years of training. This is where weight training becomes psychological; focus and control play a large role. It can take years of training for some individuals, before they are able to properly focus their mind enough to feel the muscles they are trying to work using various angles. Those who are just starting out usually fail to realize that in order to train the chest fully and allow for growth and development, the muscles that support the movements needed to train the chest also need to be given the same attention when it comes to development. The primary muscles supporting chest training are your triceps and anterior deltoids (front shoulder). Your upper back and your core (abs/obliques) also play a role in development.

Remember, your body is one large mass of energy and matter that is connected. Your chest is not a separate entity from any other part of your body. If you are having a problem developing a certain area, it could be that you are neglecting others. Chest is considered a multijoint movement and requires the control and flexion of a large amount of muscle groups, not just the chest, which is why knowing how to train every muscle in your body is imperative to an overall great physique in general. You cannot develop your chest properly by going to the gym and training only your chest every day. If you want a great chest, you need to learn how to have great triceps and shoulders too.

FUNDAMENTAL EXERCISES FOR BEGINNING CHEST DEVELOPMENT

Flat Bench Press

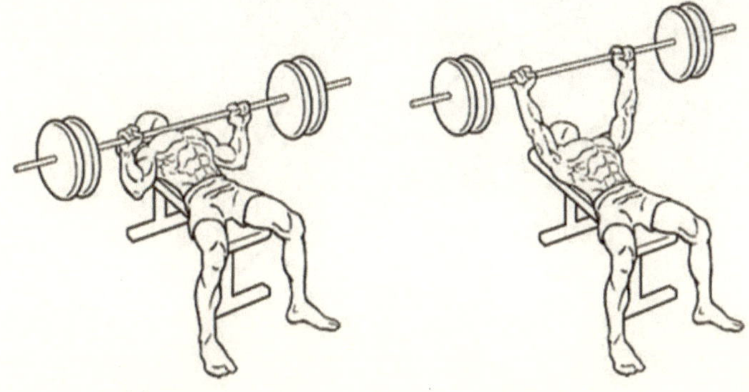

Incline Bench Press

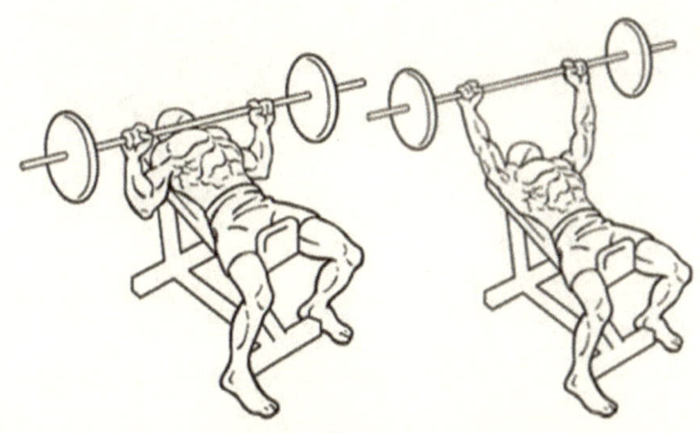

Flat/Incline Dumbbell Press

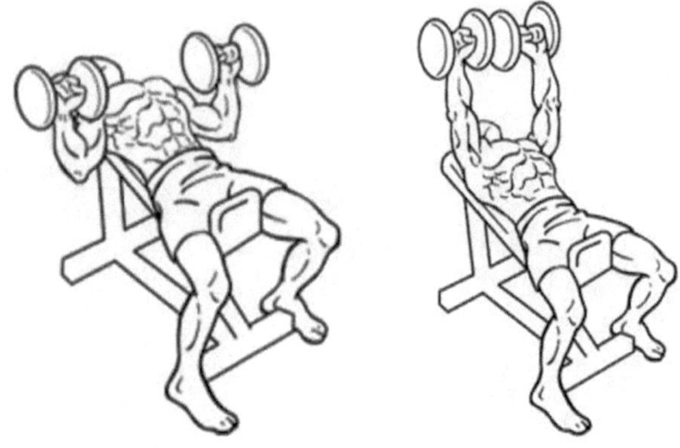

Flat/Incline Chest Flies

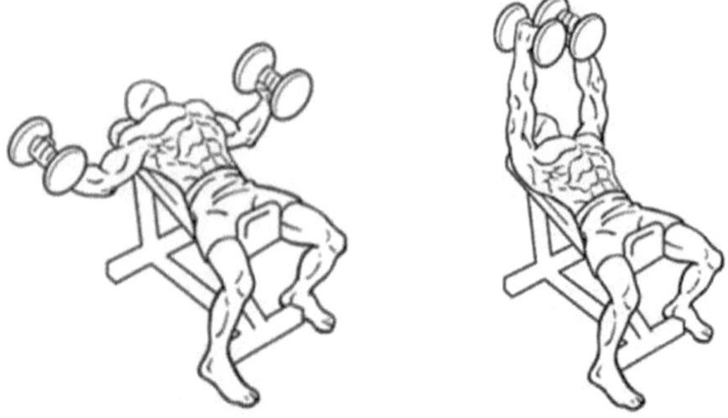

Shoulders—Your shoulders or *deltoids* consist of three main muscles: anterior (front), medial (side), and posterior (rear). All three of these need tender, sweet love to grow. Some people choose to work the trapezius muscles on shoulder day, which I do as well, though they are really more a part of the upper back than they are shoulder. Those artistic lines you see in the shoulders of people who are very lean are derived from working all three heads of the deltoid. Shoulders can be a very intimidating feature when developed properly, but they are a very delicate, and in comparison, a very weak muscle group. Getting a good shoulder workout really doesn't require that much weight at all. You will find that your medial and posterior deltoids are two of the weakest muscles in your body. The anterior deltoid is substantially stronger than the latter but still requires a great deal of safety when being utilized, either directly or as a secondary muscle in compounded movements. Working shoulders should be done with very strict form and with as much stability conscientiousness as possible. Again, start light and work your way up.

Shoulders are not a muscle group you want to take any risks with. If you aren't sure you can handle a weight, don't attempt it. Always start with the lightest weight available if you have never attempted the exercise. Get the movement correct, and then use slight increments from there. I find my posterior deltoids to be the hardest muscle to get that mind-muscle connection with. They are a very small muscle to target and require very little weight to work out when compared to the other muscles in the body. Even after years of training, it still takes me a couple of repetitions before I lock in on them, no matter what exercise I am doing. Medial deltoids are easier to target but still are a very week muscle group. No one needs to or can utilize a large amount of weight. I think the highest weight I have ever used on this exercise would be around thirty-five- to forty-pound dumbbells. And at that weight, I'm sure my form was far from perfect. Now I utilize mostly the ten- to thirty-pound ones. If you walk into a gym and you watch the most ripped guy do his lateral raises, I guarantee you they won't be heavy. If you feel silly or think you are weak doing lateral raises with fifteen-pound dumbbells, don't. Anyone who knows what they are doing won't bat an eye. These exercises can also be done on the cable machine as well, which can be helpful in finding the angle you need to achieve to target them properly.

FUNDAMENTAL EXERCISES FOR BEGINNING SHOULDER TRAINING

Seated Dumbbell Overhead Press

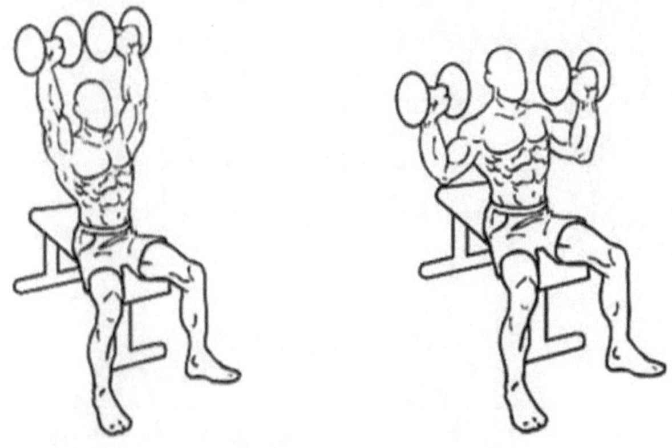

Military Press (preferably the straight-back chair)

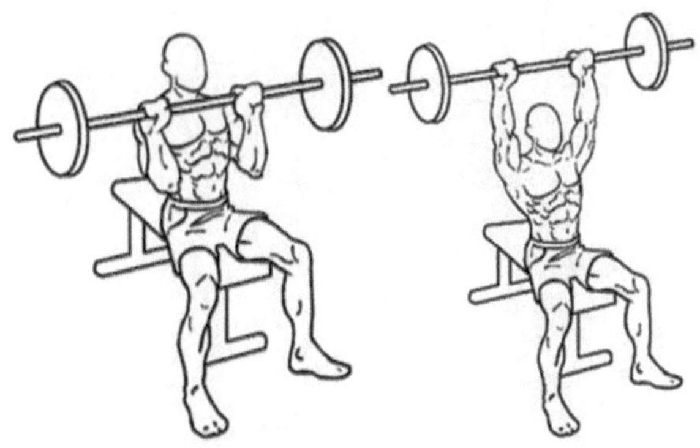

Lateral Raises

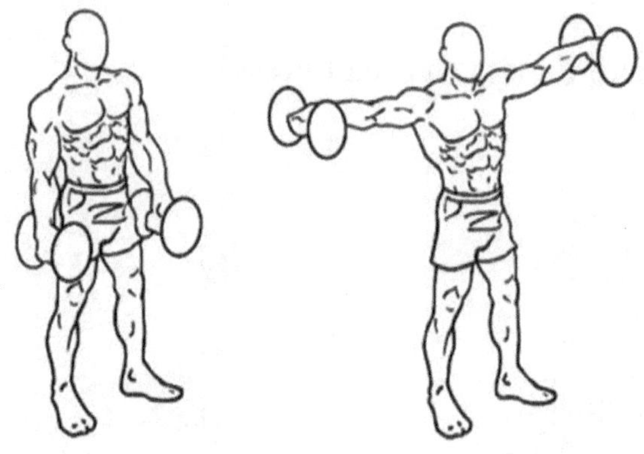

Shrugs

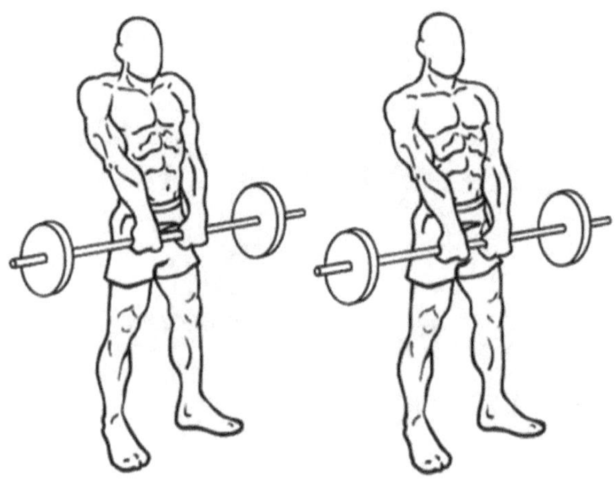

Front Raises

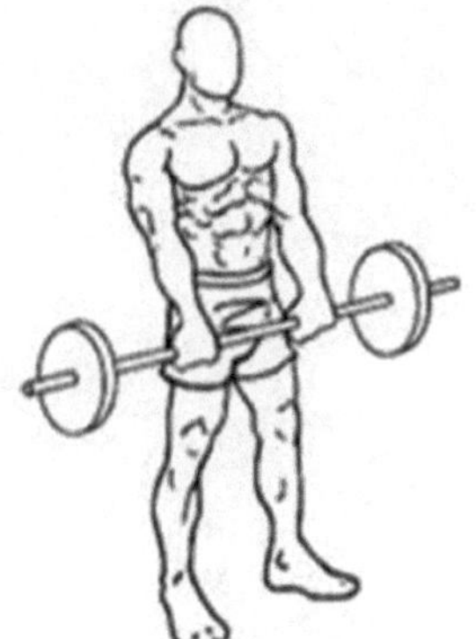 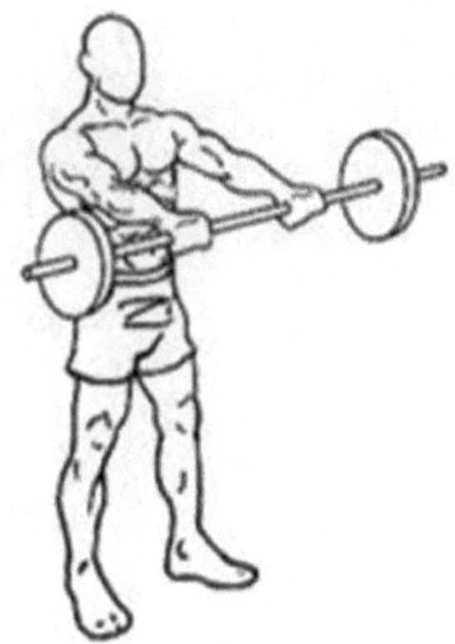

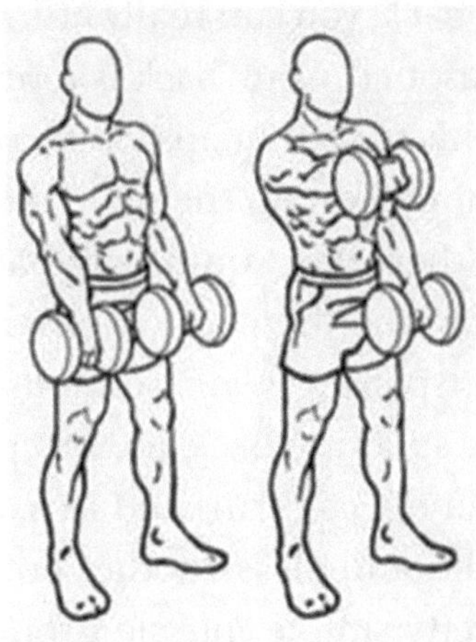

Bent-Over Flies (Cable and Dumbbell)

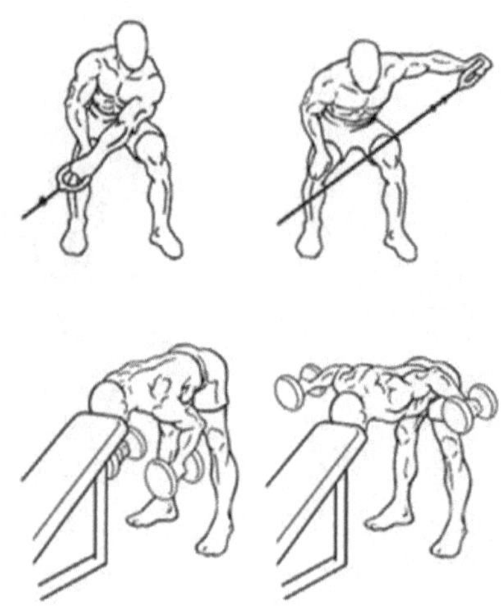

Back—For your back, you can really utilize a lot of weight once you get seasoned. Your back is a very large muscle group, second only to your quads. Some people really enjoy doing back and chest on the same day or as part of a "split," which is where you would work back and chest together on one day and then do two other muscle groups on another day, splitting your workouts into pairs. My personal favorite splits are back and biceps, chest and triceps, shoulders and legs. Arms and legs, back and chest, shoulders and abdominals is another one I have used.

Back is a pretty simple muscle group to work. The key point is to keep your spine straight. In other words, do not round your back while bending over as if you were an old man with a cane. If you are, good for you for picking up this book. Spine straight and shoulders back with your chest out like you are trying to intimidate a gorilla. That structured form will be utilized for all back exercises and most exercises in general. Again, it is very hard to explain on paper. A visual aid is most helpful. At first, some people are very hesitant to really commit to a solid back workout routine, since they feel it is silly to spend so much time working a part of their body they don't even see most of the time. But regardless of how amazing a great set of lat muscles looks when you are lean in the midsection, the development of the large muscles in the back is vital to the overall growth of the rest of your body. The back is the antagonist of the chest. That means that when you are lowering that bar on the bench press, your back muscles play a large role in the support. If your back is weak, your chest is equally weak. You can't expect your bench press to increase if you are neglecting your back muscles. The hardest of these exercises will be pull-ups. Many times people just starting out are unable to do a single one. One trick that I used to build up to even doing just one is to get a box or a bench and place it under the pull-up bar. Stand on the box or the bench, grab the bar in the up position, and slowly lower yourself down. Go as slowly as possible. Do that for three sets of eight repetitions every day you enter the gym, regardless of what muscle group you are doing. Before you start every day, attempt to do one fully. Continue to do that every day, and you *will* very quickly find you will be able to start doing one, then two, then three, and so on. Once you get up to doing three sets of twelve repetitions, add weight. Either hold a dumbbell between your ankles or strap on a weighted belt. This is the best overall exercise for lat development I have found.

Bent-Over Row/T-Bar Rows

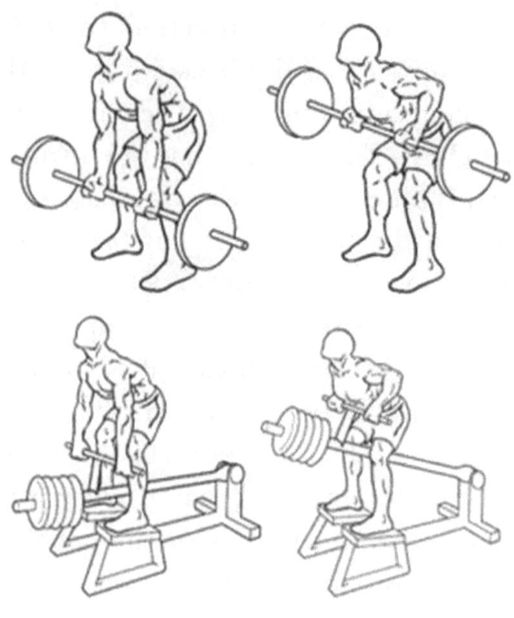

Seated Cable Row (close grip shown)

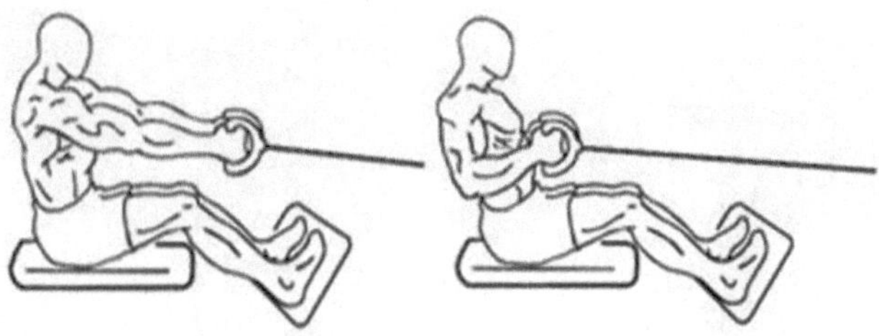

Lat Pulldown (reverse grip)

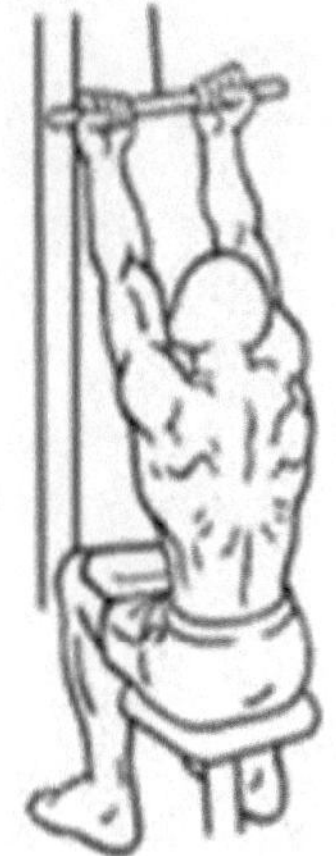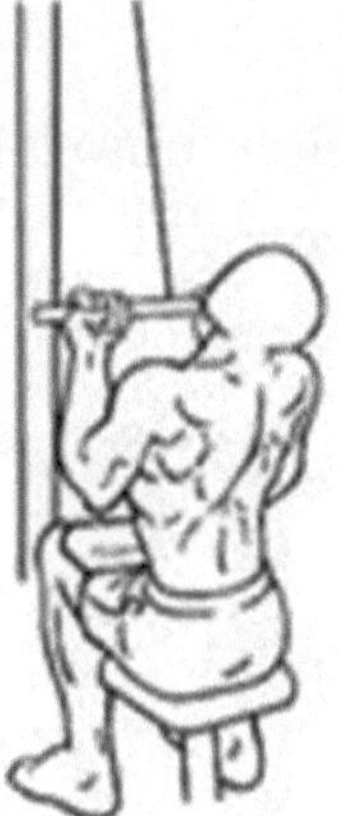

Pullups (unweighted shown)

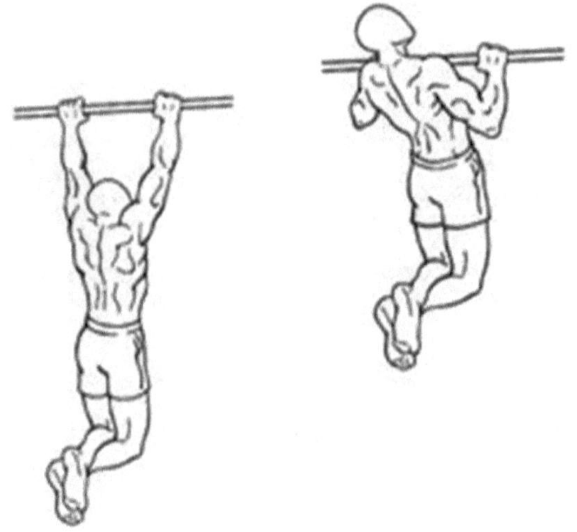

Back Extension (unweighted shown)

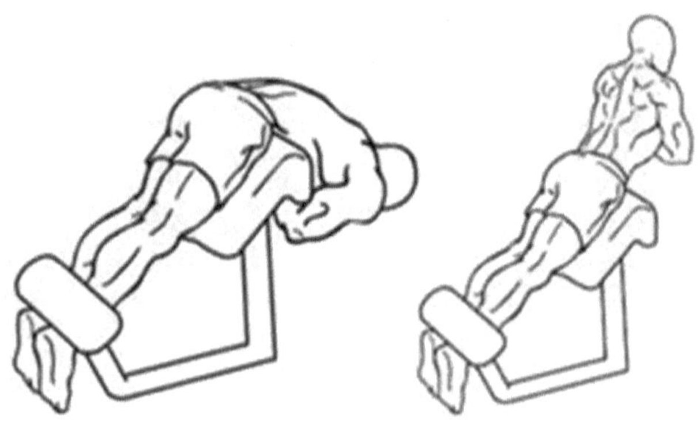

Biceps—Another one of everyone's favorites, unfortunately this one is overhyped, in my opinion. I very much like a good bicep workout. Few things feel better than leaving the gym feeling like you have grapefruits surgically implanted in your upper arms. However, your arms will look much bigger and fuller from working your triceps. It is a common misconception with newcomers that bicep curls will make your arms big, but they only encompass a quarter of your upper-arm area. The tricep makes up the other three-quarters. If you are genetically gifted with nice biceps, good for you, but if you are not, chances are, yours are not going to look very impressive unless you drop your body fat down quite a bit, because they are a pretty small muscle. But make no mistake—they are a very important muscle to strengthen.

Developing a strong pair of biceps will be essential to your overall training by way of secondary power for your back routine. Biceps also have major role to play in pulling weight toward your body, like in a lat pulldown or an upright row. Just make sure when you are working your arms, your triceps get equal focus. The preacher-curl bench will allow you to move a heavy amount of weight under strict form. Seated dumbbell curls in the incline position will allow your arms to hang slightly behind your body and make the exercise harder buy providing more isolation. It is a good idea to have at least one bicep exercise in your routine where the arms are behind the body instead of always parallel with it. Reverse-grip curls allow for the full extension of the bicep and really improve strength in the forearms at the same time.

Preacher Curl

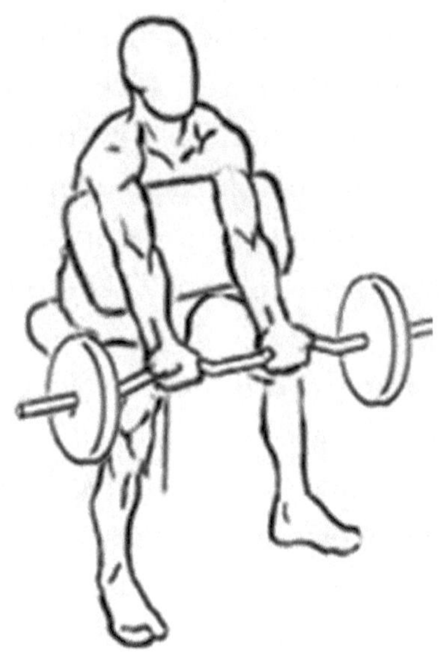

Standing Barbell Curls

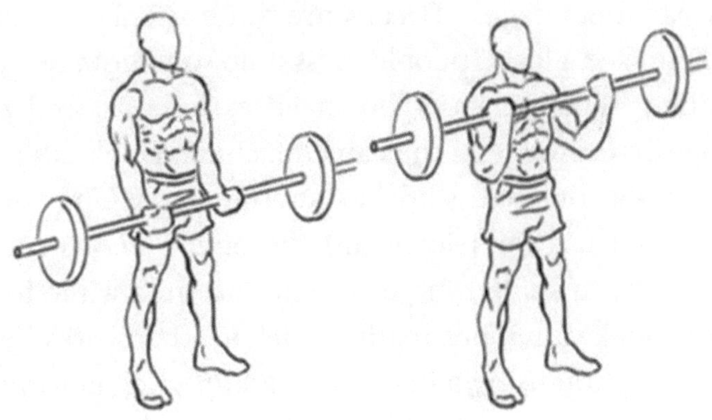

Seated Incline Dumbbell Curl

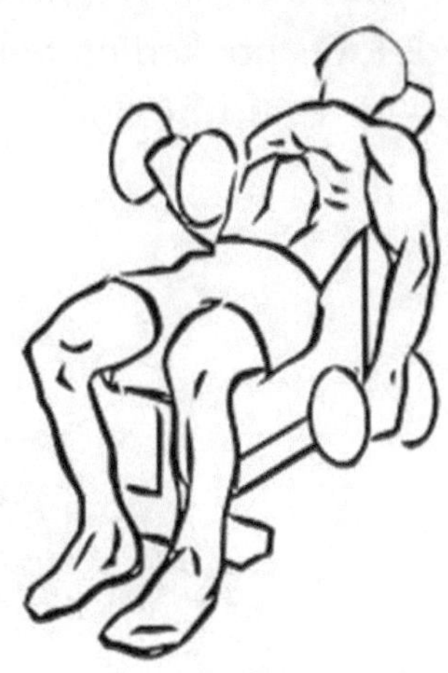

Triceps—If you want impressive arms, focus on your triceps. Heavy tricep work will make your arms grow to godlike appendages. Triceps are quite simple to work, though I see a lot of people mess it up somehow, usually by doing skull crushers, overhead extensions, and not using correct form on the cable machine. Don't fall into this; study someone who has awesome tris. The three exercises I use for triceps are the ones I *always* use. I may throw in something different once in a while for a bit of shock value, but really, I stick to what works best. The tricep dip using a bench and adding weight to your lap is *by far* the best tricep exercise when done correctly. This exercise promoted the first compliment on my arms that I received from a girl. It was high school, and I had been doing this exercise for about three months when it happened. I was hooked on bodybuilding from that day forward—for health reasons, of course.

Bench Dips

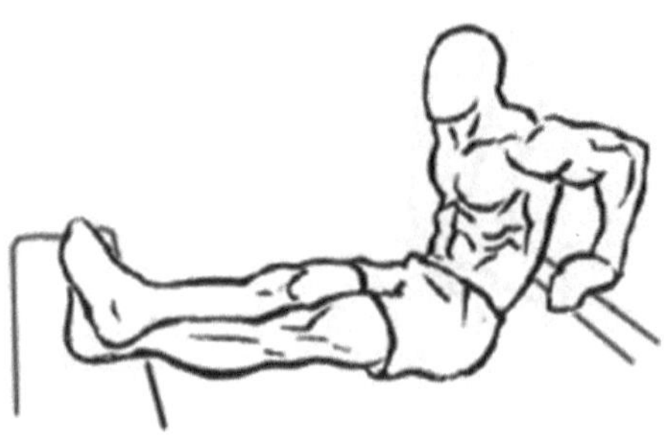

Tricep Cable Extensions

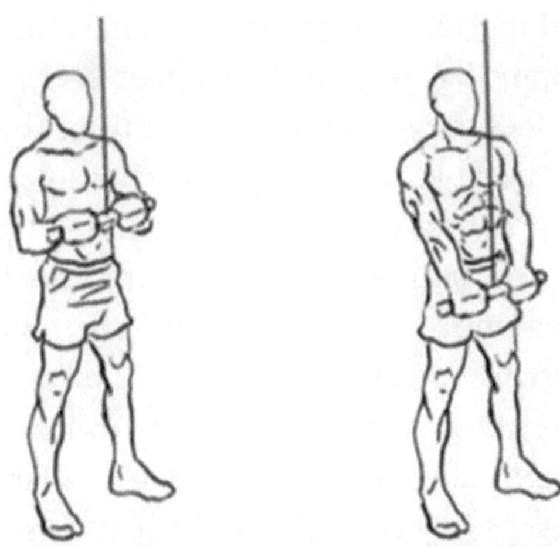

Close-Grip Incline or Decline Bench Press (flat bench shown)

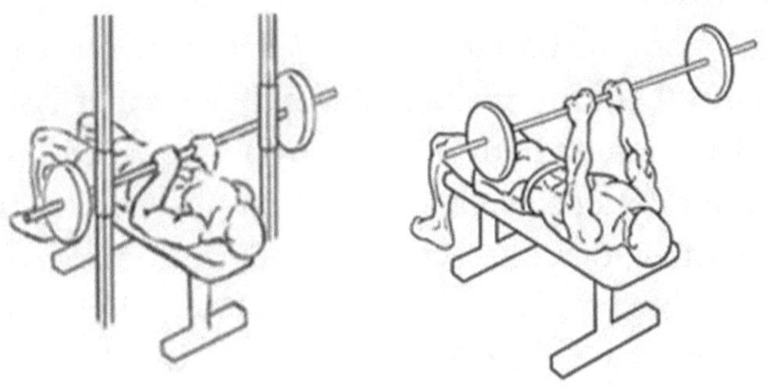

Legs—Unless you are one of those rare freaks out there who actually enjoys training your legs, chances are you aren't looking forward to this section. Most guys start out only wanting to train their upper body, since that's where we feel the sexiness lives. Truth of the matter is, you won't be able to develop much of an upper body without a good solid base to work on. As I have stated a few times now, you *must* develop your entire body if you want to maximize growth! Not only that, but your legs are 50 percent of your body mass. They make up your entire lower body. If you are looking to lose fat and get ripped, training your lower body burns a large number of calories. Heavy deadlifts and squats are two of the most taxing movements you can put on your central nervous system. Taking those movements to failure can make you feel like you've already put the down payment on the farm with sets one and two, and the closing date is set three.

I do not recommend doing deadlifts for barbell squats for beginners, since they have a greater risk potential for injury than other exercises. I would recommend not doing them alone the first time you try them and finding someone who can instruct and coach you properly before you do them under moderate load. Trying them with just the bar or with a very light kettle bell is a good place to start if you insist on attempting the movements alone. Deadlifts can also be considered a lower-back and hip exercise, but I'm going to put it in here for hamstrings. Really, they work your entire body, which is why they are so exhausting. There are different types, Romanian or stiff-legged deadlifts and regular deadlifts. The first one involves not bending your knees into a squatlike position when you lower the weight, and the other one does. Thought this exercise can be very beneficial, it is not necessary to get great lower-back and hamstring growth, though it does help tremendously to build overall strength. It can be replaced with others like the hamstring curl machine, lunges/farmer's walk, rack pulls, and weighted hyperextensions. For your quads, the master of all exercises is the barbell squat. However, this exercise can cause injury for a lot of people if not done correctly. It is best to be instructed in person, by a trainer, the first time you do them.

This exercise can also be replaced with a variety of other exercises in the gym, such as the hack-squat machine, the leg press, and other machines your gym may have that offer variations. Doing barbell squats is not the only way to get an awesome quad workout. A staple machine for working quads is the leg-extension machine. It can be used to really develop that sweet teardrop shape on the top of your knee. The leg extension is an awesome alternate angle to growing those tree trunks. Last but not least, calves—not the most exciting part of the body to work, but having little chicken legs will only take away from your overall physique, so get them growing by doing the standing calf raise machine and the seated calf machine. Weighted step-ups are also a good option, but the first two done right should be more than enough to get those twigs to grow into logs. Make sure you are using the same basic movements with your legs as you would with chest or arms. Allow the muscle to stretch at the bottom, and squeeze the contraction at the top of the exercise. Move slowly in a controlled manner. Do not bounce or do half reps. Half reps will only get you half the size.

RECOMMENDATIONS FOR STARTING LEG GROWTH

Barbell Squat

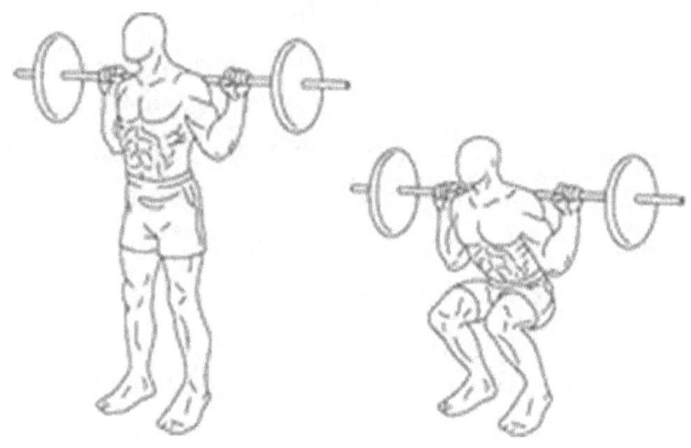

Leg Press

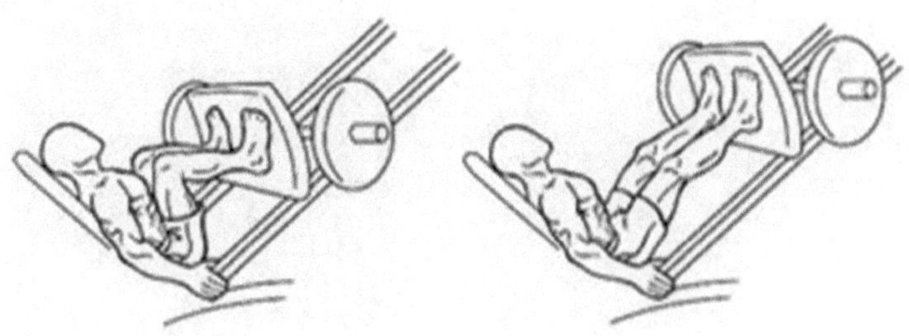

Leg Extension

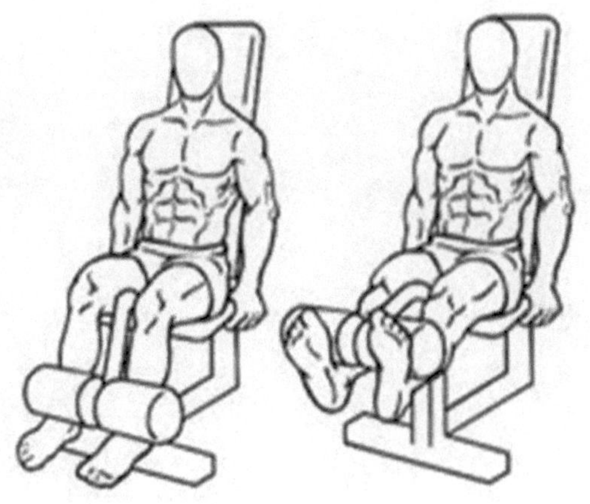

Hamstring Curls

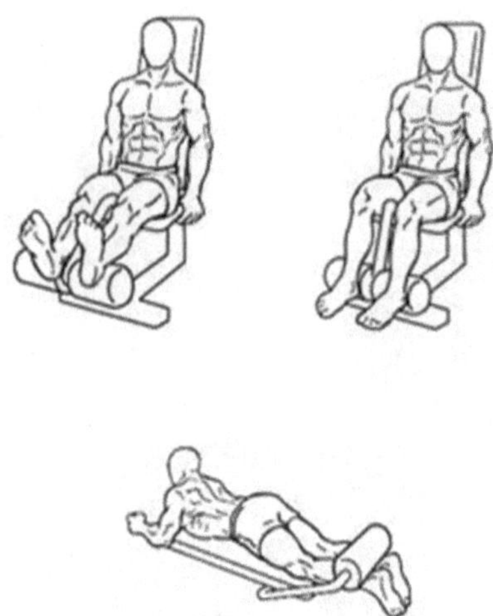

Calf Raises

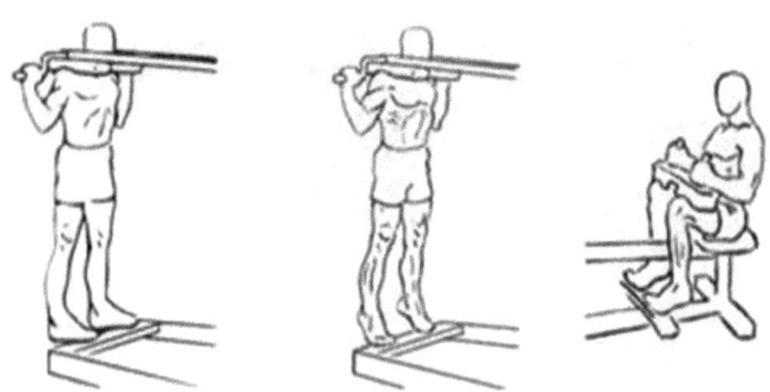

Abdominals—Ab work can seem like a real chore when you first start out. If you have a higher percentage of body fat, the only way you will ever see your efforts will be to drop enough fat to make your abs visible. You will never be able to do enough crunches or Russian twists to make those abs appear through a layer of fat on your torso. Diet is the only way. But that doesn't mean you shouldn't start working on them. If you start working on your abs when you start your journey, by the time you get to the end, where you have mastered your diet discipline and perfected an effective and efficient workout routine, it will be like pulling the cover off a Lamborghini. You can carve your abs under your temporary covering, and when the time is right, a work of art will be revealed. You must trust that the movements you are doing are creating a masterpiece that has yet to be revealed to the world. To have an effective ab routine, you don't have to spend hours working them. They can be done quickly, after your other routines. An effective ab routine can easily be done in fifteen minutes. Go to failure with every set. Your abs are fast-twitch muscles; that means that they can be worked quite frequently, and they recover quickly. If you are just starting out, they won't feel like they recover quickly. They will be quite sore for a couple of days after your first session. I have a personal ab routine I have developed, but it is unnecessary to share here. Just make sure you work your abdominals and include upper ab, lower ab and oblique exercises for a well-developed torso.

Don't be afraid to push yourself to your limits. If you are first starting out, you won't be able to go too hard the first few weeks. You will be sore as hell for about three days after your workouts until your muscles adjust. One day a week for the first three weeks may be best when you are first starting out. Muscle pain can last for several days after starting weight training. Allow yourself to experience the soreness. If you are consistent with your workouts, soon the pain will be very mild, if it occurs at all. Soon you will love the slight soreness in your muscles the next day, since you know that means you hit them good. If it means going to the washroom to puke or having to sit down with your head between your legs and cutting your workout a bit short, it's good to test your limits once you start to get comfortable. Don't listen to people who talk about stunting growth by so-called "overtraining." The majority of people who are worried about overtraining are the ones you will see not make any progress in the gym, despite going for years. It is simply an excuse not to work out. Use common sense; if you are seriously sore in one area, it's likely not a good idea to work that muscle group out at maximum weight the next day, but if you think you can't work a muscle group out more than once a week, that is completely false. As long as you are not feeling joint pain or serious fatigue, you can keep working all you want.

There are often times when I'm in the gym seven days a week. There are many times when I go twice in one day. Those days, I will adjust my carbohydrate and overall calorie intake a bit higher, but there is definitely no reason why if you are feeling well, you can't do it. It is generally good to have at least forty-eight hours between working muscle groups, to allow proper recovery, which is why my current split looks something like this. We grow stronger in life from failure if we embrace it and understand it. The same can be said for muscular development. Train to failure. Take your body to its limits and force it to rebuild stronger and better every day. Persist in your struggle, and one day you will wake up to find yourself a success.

Week One:
Monday: Shoulders/legs/abs
Tuesday: Back/biceps/cardio
Wednesday: Chest/triceps/abs/cardio
Thursday: Shoulders/legs/abs
Friday: Back/biceps/cardio
Saturday: Rest
Sunday: Rest (optional)
Chest is at rest this week

Week Two:
Monday: Chest/triceps/abs/cardio
Tuesday: Shoulders/legs/abs
Wednesday: Back/biceps/cardio
Thursday: Chest/triceps/abs/cardio
Friday: Shoulders/legs/abs
Saturday: Rest
Sunday: Rest (optional)
Back is at rest this week

Week Three:
Monday: Back/biceps/cardio
Tuesday: Chest/triceps/abs/cardio
Wednesday: Shoulders/legs/abs
Thursday: Back/biceps/cardio
Friday: Chest/triceps/abs/cardio

Saturday: Rest
Sunday: Rest (optional)
Shoulders are at rest this week

If you are using the weekends as your rest days, on Monday just continue on the rotation of muscle groups. That way, each muscle group gets two workouts per week for a three-week period, with one of the muscle groups having just one workout per week for rest purposes. If you miss a day during the week, then you can just continue on the rotation through the muscle groups your next day in or use a Saturday or Sunday to catch up. Abs and cardio can be fit in anywhere you like. This is just what I do. Abs and cardio can be done daily if you have enough energy and aren't too sore. To save time, they also don't need to be done in the gym. But as with anything, don't overdo it. If you are burning too many calories doing cardio, your energy systems may give out on you toward the end of your week. You want to keep it all in moderation and expend your food energy consistently, the same energy toward each activity you are doing. One tip I have found helped me a lot is to make sure you get a good session of HIIT cardio in the day of or the day after your cheat day.

You have now furthered your knowledge of how to start building yourself into a Greek god. Again, this is just a brief read on the basic exercises you will need to learn fully for the best result on your journey. This is not meant to be personal-training advice. Success will not come by reading this alone; you need proper visual instruction on how to perform these exercises. Then get yourself into the gym and start experimenting with your body. These are muscle groups and foundation exercises you want to focus on. There are many exercises, hundreds in fact, for each muscle, however, these are the foundation exercises that all professional body-builders base their routines around. They may add variances, with different angles, benches and cables, but all they are doing is mimicking these fundamental exercises using a variety of machines and equipment.

This book is meant to help convince you of your potential. It is written with hopes that it can help at least some people realize that they have greatness within them. I'm not sure how I brought myself to make that life-changing alteration that one day, when I just decided I had had enough of not doing what I knew I had the potential to do. I can't pinpoint the influence that made me flip that switch to start taking control of my mind and my thoughts. I'm not sure what guided me to start being in control of my life and how I went about it in my own way, no longer listening to outside influence, no longer making choices based on the opinions of other people. I set out what I wanted from life and started to work toward that every day with focus. That's the reason I want to put this experience in writing. I don't know what that spark was for me, but it had to be influenced some way. Something resonated in my mind with what I was experiencing in my life and set me on this path I am on. I am hoping that this book may be that spark someone else needs to make that leap of faith and go for what they truly desire in life.

Best wishes,
Robert

ABOUT THE AUTHOR

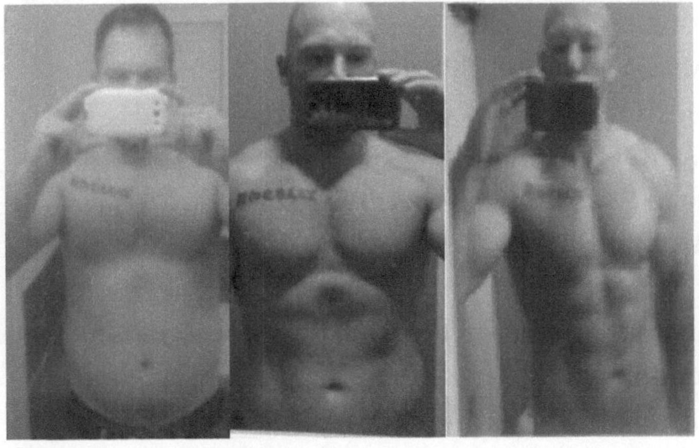

ROBERT GRANT IS a certified personal trainer and fitness enthusiast. His philosophy of training is to strengthen the mind as well as improve the aesthetics of the body.

A lover of music and traveling, Grant defines himself by his character and firmly believes even small acts of kindness can change the world. It is his hope that *Muscle Mind* offers others a chance to learn and grow from his experiences.

Alcohol and the Male Reproductive System
Mary Ann Emanuele, M.D., and Nicholas Emanuele, M.D.
https://pubs.niaaa.nih.gov/publications/arh25-4/282-287.htm

Am J Public Health. 2016 September; 106(9): 1586–1591. Published online 2016 September. doi: 10.2105/AJPH.2016.303336
PMCID: PMC4981808
Key findings on Alcohol Consumption and a Variety of Health Outcomes From the Nurses' Health Study
https://www.ncbi.nlm.nih.gov/pmc/articles/PMC4981808/1

Adverse effects of creatine supplementation: fact or fiction?
Poortmans JR[1], Francaux M.
Author information
1
Physiological Chemistry, Higher Institute of Physical Education and Readaptation, Free University of Brussels, Bruxelles, Belgium. jrpoortm@ulb.ac.be
https://www.ncbi.nlm.nih.gov/pubmed/10999421

Med Sci Sports Exerc. 2000 Feb;32(2):291-6.

Acute creatine loading increases fat-free mass, but does not affect blood pressure, plasma creatinine, or CK activity in men and women.

Mihic S[1], MacDonald JR, McKenzie S, Tarnopolsky MA.

Author information

1

Department of Kinesiology, McMaster University, Hamilton, Ontario, Canada.

https://www.ncbi.nlm.nih.gov/pubmed/10694109

J Pain Res. 2016; 9: 735–744.

Published online 2016 Sep 30. doi: 10.2147/JPR.S98182

PMCID: PMC5053383

Medical cannabis – the Canadian perspective

Gordon D Ko,[1,2] Sara L Bober,[1] Sean Mindra,[3] and Jason M Moreau[1]

[1]Apollo Applied Research Inc.

[2]Department of Medicine, Sunnybrook Health Sciences Centre, University of Toronto, Toronto

[3]University of Ottawa Medical School, Ottawa, ON, Canada

Correspondence: Gordon D Ko, Apollo Applied Research Inc., 201-240 Duncan Mill Road, Toronto, ON M3B 3S6, Canada, Email moc.prpokrd@naej

Author information ▼ Copyright and License information ▼

Medical Press Limited, provided the work is properly attributed.
https://www.ncbi.nlm.nih.gov/pmc/articles/PMC5053383/

Future Med Chem. Author manuscript; available in PMC 2010 Aug 1.
Published in final edited form as:
Future Med Chem. 2009 Oct; 1(7): 1333–1349.
doi: 10.4155/fmc.09.93
PMCID: PMC2828614
NIHMSID: NIHMS155268

Cannabinoids as novel anti-inflammatory drugs

Prakash Nagarkatti,[†] Rupal Pandey,[*] Sadiye Amcaoglu Rieder,[*] Venkatesh L Hegde, and Mitzi Nagarkatti

[†] Author for correspondence: Department of Pathology, Microbiology and Immunology, University of South Carolina, School of Medicine, Columbia, SC 29208, USA, ude.cs.demcsu@kraganp

[*]Both authors contributed equally to this review

Author information ▼ Copyright and License information

https://www.ncbi.nlm.nih.gov/pmc/articles/PMC2828614/

J Zhejiang Univ Sci. 2003 Mar-Apr;4(2):236-40.

A research on the relationship between ejaculation and serum testosterone level in men.

Jiang M[1], Xin J, Zou Q, Shen JW.

Author information

1

Department of Life Science, Hangzhou Normal College, Hangzhou 310020, China. jiangmy@mail.hz.zj.cn
https://www.ncbi.nlm.nih.gov/pubmed/12659241?dopt=Abstract

World J Urol. 2001 Nov;19(5):377-82.
Endocrine response to masturbation-induced orgasm in healthy men following a 3-week sexual abstinence.
Exton MS[1], Krüger TH, Bursch N, Haake P, Knapp W, Schedlowski M, Hartmann U.
Author information
1
Institut für Medizinische Psychologie, Universitätsklinikum Essen, Germany. michael.exton@uni-essen.de
https://www.ncbi.nlm.nih.gov/pubmed/11760788?dopt=Abstract

Free Radic Biol Med. Author manuscript; available in PMC 2008 Mar 1.

Published in final edited form as:

Free Radic Biol Med. 2007 Mar 1; 42(5): 665–674.

Published online 2006 Dec 14. doi: 10.1016/j.freeradbiomed.2006.12.005

PMCID: PMC1859864

NIHMSID: NIHMS19360

Alternate Day Calorie Restriction Improves Clinical Findings and Reduces Markers of Oxidative Stress and Inflammation in Overweight Adults with Moderate Asthma

James B. Johnson,[1,*] Warren Summer,[2] Roy G. Cutler,[3] Bronwen Martin,[3] Dong-Hoon Hyun,[3] Vishwa D. Dixit,[4] Michelle Pearson,[3] Matthew Nassar,[3] Stuart Maudsley,[3] Olga Carlson,[5] Sujit John,[6] Donald R. Laub,[7] and Mark P. Mattson[3]

[1] Department of Surgery, Louisiana State University Medical Center, New Orleans, LA

[2] Department of Pulmonary Medicine, Louisiana State University Medical Center, New Orleans, LA

[3] Laboratory of Neurosciences, National Institute on Aging Intramural Research Program, Baltimore, MD

[4] Laboratory of Immunology, National Institute on Aging Intramural Research Program, Baltimore, MD

[5] Diabetes Section, National Institute on Aging Intramural Research Program, Baltimore, MD

[6] Deparment of Mathematics, University of New Orleans, New Orleans, LA

[7] Department of Surgery, Stanford University, Palo Alto, CA

*Correspondence: James B. Johnson, https://www.ncbi.nlm.nih.gov/pmc/articles/PMC1859864/

Int J Health Sci (Qassim). 2014 Jul; 8(3): V–VI.
PMCID: PMC4257368

Role of Intermittent Fasting on Improving Health and Reducing Diseases

Salah Mesalhy Aly, Ph.D.

Prof. of Pathology & Head of Med. Labs Dept, Faculty of Applied Medical Sciences, Editor, International Journal of Health Sciences, Qassim University, KSA. Email: moc. liamtoh@ylahalaS

https://www.ncbi.nlm.nih.gov/pmc/articles/PMC4257368/

World J Diabetes. 2017 Apr 15; 8(4): 154–164.
Published online 2017 Apr 15. doi: 10.4239/wjd.v8.i4.154
PMCID: PMC5394735

Effects of intermittent fasting on health markers in those with type 2 diabetes: A pilot study

Terra G Arnason, Matthew W Bowen, and Kerry D Mansell

Terra G Arnason, Department of Medicine, College of Medicine, University of Saskatchewan, Saskatoon, SK S7K 5E5, Canada

Matthew W Bowen, Kerry D Mansell, Division of Pharmacy, College of Pharmacy and Nutrition, University of Saskatchewan, Saskatoon, SK S7K 5E5, Canada

Author contributions: Arnason TG and Mansell KD contributed equally to this work; Arnason TG and Mansell KD designed the research; Bowen MW performed the research, designed the analytical tools and analysed the data; Arnason TG and Mansell KD wrote the paper.

Correspondence to: Kerry D Mansell, BSP, PharmD, MBA, Associate Professor, Division of Pharmacy, College of Pharmacy and Nutrition, University of Saskatchewan, 104 Clinic Place, Saskatoon, SK S7K 5E5, Canada. ac.ksasu@llesnam.yrrek

Telephone: +1-306-9665235 Fax: +1-306-9666377

Author information ▼ Article notes ► Copyright and License information ►

https://www.ncbi.nlm.nih.gov/pmc/articles/
PMC5394735/

2017

- Recycling of iron via autophagy is critical for the transition from glycolytic to respiratory growth
  Horie T, Kawamata T, Matsunami M, Ohsumi Y.
  J. Biol. Chem., 10.1074/jbc.M116.762963, [Faculty of 1000], *in press*
- Zinc starvation induces autophagy in yeast
  Kawamata T, Horie T, Matsunami M, Sasaki M, Ohsumi Y.
  J. Biol. Chem., 10.1074/jbc.M116.762948, [editor's pick up], *in press*

2016

- The intrinsically disordered protein Atg13 mediates supramolecular assembly of autophagy initiation complexes
  Yamamoto H, Fujioka Y, Suzuki SW, Noshiro D, Suzuki H, Kondo-Kakuta C, Kimura Y, Hirano H, Ando T, Noda NN & Ohsumi Y
  Dev. Cell., 2016, 38, 86-99.
- Structural basis for receptor-mediated selective autophagy of aminopeptidase I aggregates

Yamasaki A, Watanabe Y, Adachi W, Suzuki K, Matoba K, Kirisako H, Kumeta H, Nakatogawa H, Ohsumi Y, Inagaki F, Noda NN*
Cell Rep., 2016, 16, 19-27.

http://www.ohsumilab.aro.iri.titech.ac.jp/publication.html

Finally making sense of the double-slit experiment
Yakir Aharonov,[a,b,c,1] Eliahu Cohen,[d,1,2] Fabrizio Colombo,[e] Tomer Landsberger,[c,2] Irene Sabadini,[e] Daniele C. Struppa,[a,b] and Jeff Tollaksen[a,b]
[a]Institute for Quantum Studies, Chapman University, Orange, CA, 92866;
[b]Schmid College of Science and Technology, Chapman University, Orange, CA, 92866;
[c]School of Physics and Astronomy, Tel Aviv University, Tel Aviv 6997801, Israel;
[d]H. H. Wills Physics Laboratory, University of Bristol, Bristol BS8 1TL, United Kingdom;
[e]Dipartimento di Matematica, Politecnico di Milano, 9 20133 Milan, Italy
[1]To whom correspondence may be addressed. Email: ude.nampahc@vonoraha and ku.ca.lotsirb@nehoc.uhaile.
Contributed by Yakir Aharonov, March 20, 2017 (sent for review September 26, 2016; reviewed by Pawel Mazur and Neil Turok)

Author contributions: Y.A. conceived research; Y.A., E.C., and T.L. designed research; Y.A., E.C., F.C., T.L., I.S., D.C.S., and J.T. performed research; and E.C., T.L., and J.T. wrote the paper.
Reviewers: P.M., University of South Carolina; and N.T., Perimeter Institute.
[2]E.C. and T.L. contributed equally to this work.

Arntz, William, Betsy Chasse, Mark Vicente, Marlee Matlin, Elaine Hendrix, and Barry Newman. *What the Bleep!?: Down the Rabbit Hole.* , 2014.

Hill, Napoleon. *Think and Grow Rich*. New York: Fawcett Books, 1987. Print.

Gikandi, David C. *Happy Pocket Full of Money: Infinite Wealth and Abundance in the Here and Now*. Place of publication not identified: Hampton Roads Pub Co Inc, 2015. Internet resource.

Wattles, W D, and Diana Majlinger. *The Science of Getting Rich.* , 2017. Internet resource.

Byrne, Rhonda. *The Secret*. New York[etc.: Atria Books [etc., 2016. Print.

www.ingramcontent.com/pod-product-compliance
Lightning Source LLC
Chambersburg PA
CBHW051452250726
48655CB00001B/370